DECODING DIABETES

PROVEN WAYS FOR PREVENTION AND REMISSION OF TYPE 2 DIABETES

VISHWANATH B L

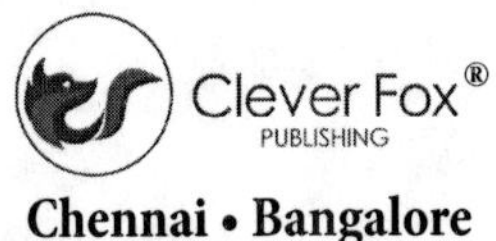

Chennai • Bangalore

CLEVER FOX PUBLISHING
Chennai, India

Published by CLEVER FOX PUBLISHING 2025

ISBN: 978-93-6707-936-2

CONTENTS

Decoding Diabetes .... *ix*
Preface .... *xi*

SECTION 1: THE TRUTH ABOUT DIABETES – FOUNDATIONS YOU WERE NEVER TOLD **1**

1. Introduction 2
2. The Silent Onset – How Diabetes Develops in the Body 6
3. Early Biomarkers to Know Diabetes and Metabolic Risk 9
4. The Hidden Damage Before Diabetes 13
5. Cracking the C-Peptide Code – What It Really Tells You About Your Diabetes 17
6. Essential test in diabetes – What to measure, what they mean? 21
7. I Feel Fine… So Why Worry? The Silent Damage of High Blood Sugar 28
8. Diabetes at 30? Why Young Indians Are Crashing Early and How to Change Course 32
9. Diabetes in Women – Unseen, Unequal, Unspoken 36
10. Skinny But Sick – India's Hidden Diabetics 40
11. The Inflammation Equation – Why Diabetes Isn't Just About Sugar 45

12. Toxic Blood Sugar – How Everyday Chemicals Disrupt Metabolism and Cause Diabetes 52
13. Digital Diabetes – How Screens, Sleep Loss, and Social Media Are Spiking Your Sugars 56

SECTION 2

1. The Turning Point – Can Diabetes Go Into Remission? 62
2. The Reversal Code – How Early Diabetes Can Be Undone Without Medications 66
3. Proven Strategies for Prevention, Remission, and Good Metabolic Health 70

SECTION 3: NEW RULES OF NUTRITION FOR BLOOD SUGAR CONTROL 74

1. Breaking Norms, Breaking Dietary Misconceptions 75
2. Low Carb Science. How Cutting Carbs Can Send Diabetes into Remission 78
3. The Power of Protein – The Missing Link in Diabetes Management 81
4. The Low-Fat Lie – Rethinking Fats in Diabetes and Metabolic Health 86
5. The Sugar That Wasn't Sweet — How Hidden Carbs Spike Your Blood Sugar 90
6. Facts vs. Fads – Do Traditional Remedies Like ACV and Methi Really Work? 96
7. Seed Oils and Sugar Spikes – The Hidden Link in Your Kitchen 99

8. Can You Eat Less and Heal More? 105
9. Fasting Safely — What Every Diabetic Must Know Before Skipping a Meal 109
10. Smart Supplementing – What Every Diabetic Should (and Shouldn't) Take 114

SECTION 4: LIFESTYLE AS A MEDICINE – DAILY ROUTINE THAT HEALS 118

1. Lifestyle Is the Lifeline – Daily Habits That Change Everything 119
2. Move Like Your Ancestors – Rediscovering Natural Exercise 124
3. Sleep, Stress & Sugar — The Unseen Axis 128
4. The Yogic Prescription – Ancient Practice, Modern Diabetes Cure 131
5. Stronger Muscles, Stronger Metabolism – Resistance Training for Diabetes Control 136
6. Running and Diabetes – Stride Smart for Better Metabolic Health 140
7. The Purpose-Driven Path to Reversing Diabetes 144

SECTION 5: DIABETES COMPANION CHAPTERS 147

1. Growing Up With Sugar – Diabetes in Adolescents and Teens 148
2. Metabolic Karma – How Childhood Habits Shape Adult Diabetes 153

3. Diabetes in the Elderly – Beyond Sugar, Beyond Pills 157
4. Sugar in the Womb – The Hidden Crisis of Gestational Diabetes 161
5. Your Liver Knows – Fatty Liver and Diabetes: Two Sides of the Same Coin 166
6. The Gut Connection – How Your Microbiome Shapes Blood Sugar and Metabolism 169
7. The New Fat Burners – Game-Changing Drugs Transforming Diabetes and Weight Loss 173
8. Monitoring Sugars in the Digital Age – Beyond Finger Pricks 181
9. The Festival Survival Guide – Enjoy Sweets Without Spiking 186
10. Diabetic Travel Hacks – Staying on Track Away From Home 189
11. Diabetes and Cognitive Decline – The Forgotten Link 193
12. Sugar, Cells, and Cancer – What Every Diabetic Should Know 197
13. The Sweet Deception – Are Diet Drinks Really Safe for Diabetics? 201
14. Sick-Day Rules for Diabetics – What to Do When Illness Strikes 206
15. Shots That Shield – Essential Vaccines for People with Diabetes 210

16. Personalized Diabetes – Future of Genomics & Biomarkers 214

SECTION 6: FINAL INSIGHTS **219**

1. The Final Word – From Knowledge to Action 220
2. Lifestyle FAQs – Diabetes in the Real World 225

DECODING DIABETES

📖 How to Read This Book

You don't have to read *Decoding Diabetes* cover to cover. Use it like a roadmap—jump to the parts that matter most to you.

- Newly Diagnosed?
  Start with Section 1 to understand what's happening inside your body.
- Want Reversal or Prevention?
  Go to Section 2 for proven remission strategies.
- Confused About Diet?
  See Section 3 for clear guidance on carbs, protein, fats, and traditional remedies.
- Ready for Lifestyle Change?
  Explore Section 4 for routines on sleep, stress, exercise, and yoga.
- In a Special Situation?
  Check Section 5 for women, teens, elderly, pregnancy, fatty liver, vaccines, or travel.
- Need Quick Answers?
  Flip to Section 6—FAQs, hacks, and action steps for real life.

💡 Look for the Doctor's Quick Recap at the end of every chapter—it's your instant checklist.

This book is your companion for every stage of diabetes—prevention, control, and reversal.

🙏 Acknowledgements

This book would not have been possible without the support and inspiration I've received along the way.

My heartfelt thanks to my patients, who continue to teach me that diabetes is about people, not just numbers.

To my wife, Dr. Khushbu Goel, for her constant encouragement and unconditional support, and to our special son, Ishan, whose courage and spirit inspire me every single day—this book is as much yours as it is mine.

I am also grateful to my family, mentors, colleagues, and the teams at Satva Clinic and Manipal Hospital Kanakapura Road for walking with me on this journey.

And to you, the reader—thank you for trusting me. Your decision to take charge of your health gives this book its true purpose.

PREFACE – 2025 EDITION

By Dr. Sanath Kumar, MD, Detroit, MI, USA

Food has always been the most fundamental of human needs. For most of human history, the lack of food was the greatest limiting factor for population growth and shaped the social and political systems that we live with even today. It is quite plausible that the evolutionary development of complex metabolic processes—such as lipogenesis (storing glucose as fat) and gluconeogenesis (creating glucose from fat and protein)—was itself nature's response to this periodic scarcity.

The industrial and green revolutions changed this equation forever. With the rise of mechanized agriculture, improved distribution, and economic growth, famines and malnutrition dramatically declined across much of the world. Ironically, this abundance has created an entirely new challenge for modern society—diseases of excess. Obesity, type 2 diabetes, and cardiovascular disease have now replaced hunger as the dominant metabolic threats.

This trend is especially visible in India, where the pendulum has swung from famine to food surplus within just a few generations. According to the latest data, India is home to more than 100 million adults living with diabetes, with the number projected to rise further in the coming decade. While medical and surgical interventions remain the backbone of diabetes care, the sharp contrast between the past era of scarcity and the current epidemic of metabolic disease reminds us that the roots of the problem lie in lifestyle and nutrition, not medication alone.

This book by Dr. Vishwanath B. L. is a thoughtful and courageous effort to address this fundamental truth. Trained as a physician in modern medicine, he has consistently emphasized the power of lifestyle modification—particularly intermittent fasting, balanced nutrition, and circadian alignment—as powerful, evidence-based tools for metabolic health and diabetes remission.

I have had the privilege of knowing Dr. Vishwanath for more than twenty years, and I can personally attest that he practices what he preaches. His disciplined lifestyle and scientific curiosity have inspired many of us to rethink our relationship with food. Under his guidance, I adopted intermittent fasting several years ago, and it remains one of the most beneficial health decisions I have made. Many of my family members have followed suit, finding similar improvements in their health and energy.

The second edition of Decoding Diabetes expands upon his earlier work with updated scientific evidence, Indian dietary insights, and practical tools for anyone seeking genuine metabolic transformation. I hope readers will approach this book with an open mind—setting aside conventional dogmas—and embrace its simple yet profound message: that food, when understood correctly, can be the most powerful medicine we possess.

— Sanath Kumar, MD

Detroit, Michigan, USA

March 2025

SECTION 1

THE TRUTH ABOUT DIABETES – FOUNDATIONS YOU WERE NEVER TOLD

CHAPTER 1

INTRODUCTION

> "Understanding diabetes is the first step toward defeating it."
>
> – **Dr. Vishwanath BL**

Diabetes is not simply a "sugar problem." It is a chronic metabolic condition in which your body struggles to manage glucose (sugar) in the bloodstream due to problems with insulin, a key hormone that regulates blood sugar.

When insulin function fails—either due to lack of production or resistance at the cellular level—glucose builds up in the blood, leading to widespread damage over time.

The 7 Types of Diabetes You Should Know

1. Type 1 Diabetes – Autoimmune destruction of insulin-producing beta cells; requires lifelong insulin.
2. Type 2 Diabetes – Caused by insulin resistance, driven by lifestyle and genetics; often reversible.
3. Gestational Diabetes Mellitus (GDM) – Develops during pregnancy; increases future risk for both mother and child.

4. Latent Autoimmune Diabetes in Adults (LADA) – "Type 1.5" diabetes; late-onset, slower progression.
5. Maturity-Onset Diabetes of the Young (MODY) – Rare genetic form diagnosed in teens or young adults.
6. Secondary Diabetes – Caused by medications, pancreatic disease, or hormonal conditions.
7. Neonatal Diabetes – Diagnosed in infants; often linked to genetic mutations.

India's Diabetes Snapshot – 2025

According to the ICMR–INDIAB study (2023, published in The Lancet):

– 101 million Indians have diabetes
– 136 million have prediabetes, many are undiagnosed
– 95%+ of cases are Type 2
– Nearly 1 in 2 people with diabetes are unaware of their condition
– Type 2 diabetes now affects Indians as early as their 30s

India now has the second-largest diabetic population in the world, after China.

Insulin: The Hormone at the Heart of It All

Insulin helps move glucose from your blood into your cells for energy. But when your cells become resistant to insulin, your body compensates by producing more of it—until the pancreas can no longer keep up. This insulin resistance silently progresses to Type 2 Diabetes.

Why Early Detection Matters

Most people develop insulin resistance years before blood sugar levels rise. During this phase, silent damage occurs to the eyes, kidneys, nerves, and the heart.

Prediabetes is not just a warning—it is already a sign of metabolic breakdown.

Diabetes Is Preventable. Often Reversible.

The encouraging truth: Type 2 Diabetes is not always a lifelong disease. With early detection and lifestyle change—diet, exercise, fasting, sleep—many individuals can put diabetes into remission without lifelong medication.

Quick Recap

- Diabetes is a group of metabolic disorders, not just one condition
- As of 2025, India has over 100 million diabetics
- Most have Type 2, often linked to poor lifestyle habits
- Prediabetes is reversible if caught early
- Modern medicine now classifies 7 distinct types of diabetes

References

1. Indian Council of Medical Research–India Diabetes (ICMR–INDIAB) Study. Lancet Diabetes & Endocrinology, 2023.
2. American Diabetes Association. Standards of Medical Care in Diabetes—2024. Diabetes Care.
3. World Health Organization. Classification of diabetes mellitus. 2019.

4. International Diabetes Federation (IDF) Diabetes Atlas, 10th edition, 2021.
5. National Institute of Diabetes and Digestive and Kidney Diseases (NIDDK), U.S. Department of Health and Human Services.

CHAPTER 2

THE SILENT ONSET – HOW DIABETES DEVELOPS IN THE BODY

The Slow Beginning: Insulin Resistance

Diabetes rarely begins overnight. It starts silently, often years before a diagnosis is made. The earliest and most crucial change in the body is the development of insulin resistance.

Insulin resistance occurs when the body's cells—particularly in the liver, muscles, and fat — stop responding effectively to insulin. As a result, glucose remains in the bloodstream instead of entering the cells. To compensate, the pancreas produces more insulin, creating a state of hyperinsulinemia.

Over time, this resistance becomes more pronounced, especially when compounded by poor lifestyle habits and excess visceral fat, particularly around the abdomen.

The Role of the Pancreas: Overworked and Exhausted

To maintain normal blood sugar levels, the pancreas increases insulin production. Initially, this compensatory response works well. However, as insulin resistance worsens over time, the pancreatic beta cells become overburdened.

Eventually, these cells begin to fail, leading to insufficient insulin production. This is the tipping point where blood sugar levels start to rise, progressing toward type 2 diabetes.

From Prediabetes to Diabetes

Prediabetes is a condition where blood glucose levels are higher than normal but not yet in the diabetic range. Most individuals with prediabetes show no symptoms, making it easy to overlook.

However, even at this stage, silent damage may already be occurring, affecting the heart, kidneys, eyes, and nerves. Without timely intervention, a large proportion of people with prediabetes go on to develop full-blown diabetes within 5 to 10 years.

Risk Factors and Triggers

Several interconnected factors contribute to insulin resistance and the eventual onset of diabetes:

- Sedentary lifestyle and lack of exercise
- Diet high in refined carbohydrates and sugar
- Poor sleep quality and duration
- Chronic stress and elevated cortisol
- Family history of diabetes

– Epigenetic changes influenced by long-term environment and habits

Addressing these modifiable risk factors early on can greatly reduce the likelihood of disease progression.

CHAPTER 3

EARLY BIOMARKERS TO KNOW DIABETES AND METABOLIC RISK

Why Biomarkers Matter

Glucose levels are often the last to change in the progression toward diabetes. Long before fasting sugar or HbA1c rise, metabolic dysfunction is already brewing. Biomarkers offer a window into these early changes, giving clinicians and individuals a chance to detect, prevent, and reverse the condition before it becomes full-blown diabetes.

Key Biomarkers to Assess Diabetes and Metabolic Risk

These biomarkers can provide early insight into metabolic dysfunction and diabetes risk:

Biomarker	Significance	Reference Range	Optimal Range
Fasting Insulin	Early marker of insulin resistance	2–25 μIU/mL	2–8 μIU/mL

HOMA-IR	Insulin resistance estimate (Insulin × Glucose ÷ 405)	<2.5	<1.5
Triglyceride/ HDL Ratio	Predictor of insulin sensitivity	<3.0	<2.0
Adiponectin	Low levels = higher resistance	4–26 µg/ mL	>10 µg/mL
hs-CRP	Inflammation marker linked to insulin resistance	<3 mg/L	<1 mg/L
Fasting Glucose	Checked after 8 hours fasting; >100 mg/dL indicates risk	70–99 mg/dL	80–90 mg/dL
HbA1c	3-month glucose average	<5.7%	5.0–5.4%
Uric Acid	Linked to insulin resistance & NAFLD	3.5–7.2 mg/dL	<5.5 mg/dL
ALT	NAFLD marker	<40 IU/L	<25 IU/L
Blood Pressure	Cardiometabolic risk factor	<140/<90 mmHg	<130/<80 mmHg
Waist Circumference	Marker of visceral fat	<102 cm (M), <88 cm (F)	<90 cm (M), <80 cm (F)
Vitamin D (25-OH)	Low vitamin D linked with insulin resistance	20–50 ng/mL	40–60 ng/mL
CGM Metrics	Real-time glycemic variability and post-meal spikes	Time in Range >70%	Time in Range >80%

How These Biomarkers Help

These tests give insights into metabolic dysfunction years before conventional blood sugar rises. They help catch problems earlier, guide lifestyle changes, and personalize diabetes prevention. CGM (Continuous Glucose Monitoring) is now a valuable tool to track real-time glucose responses to meals, stress, and sleep patterns. Low Vitamin D is also associated with increased insulin resistance and is commonly overlooked.

Who Should Get These Tests Done?

- Anyone aged "20 years or older" who is "overweight or obese"
- "All individuals above 30 years", regardless of weight, should get these tests "once a year"
- Those with "family history of diabetes", "PCOS", "fatty liver", or "chronic fatigue"
- Individuals with "central obesity", "elevated triglycerides", or "acanthosis nigricans"

Suggested Lab Panel for Indian Patients

- Fasting insulin and glucose (to calculate HOMA-IR)
- Lipid profile (Triglyceride/HDL ratio)
- hs-CRP and ALT
- Uric acid and Vitamin D (25-OH)
- Blood pressure and waist circumference
- Optional: Adiponectin (if accessible)
- CGM (for high-risk or curious individuals tracking real-time spikes)

References

1. Indian Council of Medical Research (ICMR). Standard Treatment Workflow (STW) for Type 2 Diabetes Mellitus, July 2022.
2. World Health Organization. Definition and diagnosis of diabetes mellitus and intermediate hyperglycemia, 2006.
3. American Diabetes Association. Standards of Medical Care in Diabetes—2024. Diabetes Care.
4. Means, Casey. Good Energy: The Surprising Connection Between Metabolism and Health. 2024.

CHAPTER 4

THE HIDDEN DAMAGE BEFORE DIABETES

Metabolic Dysfunction Is a Cascade, Not a Switch

Diabetes does not appear overnight. It is the final stage of a slow and silent breakdown in your body's metabolic health. Long before your blood sugar rises, your cells stop responding well to insulin, your liver accumulates fat, your pancreas works overtime, and chronic inflammation quietly damages tissues.

This phase—known as insulin resistance—often lasts for years. Ignoring it allows a metabolic domino effect to unfold, leading to diabetes and multiple organ damage.

From Warning to Damage: The Timeline of Neglect

Let's look at how the early warning signs progress if left unchecked:

Stage	What's Happening	Silent Effects
HOMA-IR >1.5	Insulin resistance begins	Weight gain, fatigue
Fasting insulin ↑	Hyperinsulinemia	PCOS, hunger, fat storage

Trig/HDL ratio ↑	High triglycerides and low HDL increase cardiovascular and diabetes risk	Fatty liver, high BP, insulin resistance
hsCRP ↑	Low-grade inflammation	Endothelial dysfunction
HbA1c 5.5–6.4%	Prediabetes	Eye, nerve, kidney damage begins

What Gets Damaged First

Even with normal blood sugar levels, key organs and systems begin to deteriorate during insulin resistance:

– "Liver": Fat accumulates, leading to NAFLD and inflammation.
– "Pancreas": Beta cells become overworked and start to fail.
– "Muscles": Reduced ability to absorb glucose, lowering metabolic flexibility.
– "Endothelium": Blood vessel linings get inflamed, raising BP and heart risk.
– "Nerves": Early signs of neuropathy, even without high sugars.

The Dangerous Misconception: "I Feel Fine"

Many people don't act because they feel healthy. But feeling fine is not the same as being metabolically healthy. The body often compensates until the burden becomes too much—by then, damage has already set in.

This lag between dysfunction and symptoms is why proactive testing and early detection matter.

Doctor's Take

By the time blood sugar rises enough to diagnose diabetes, silent damage has already taken place—often to the liver, pancreas, nerves, and blood vessels. I tell patients that the real problem isn't sugar, it's ignoring the signs that come years before it.

Why Acting Early Prevents the Domino Effect

The good news is that early insulin resistance and metabolic dysfunction are reversible. Addressing the root cause early with lifestyle changes—nutrition, movement, sleep, stress management—can halt and even reverse this domino effect.

Waiting until sugar rises means working against permanent damage. The earlier you act, the more control you have.

Quick Recap

- Diabetes develops slowly through years of metabolic dysfunction.
- Insulin resistance is the first domino—leading to fat buildup, inflammation, and beta-cell stress.
- Key organs like the liver, blood vessels, pancreas, and nerves suffer damage before blood sugar rises.
- A normal fasting sugar or HbA1c doesn't mean you're metabolically healthy.
- The earlier you act on warning signs, the more likely you are to reverse or prevent diabetes.

References

1. Indian Council of Medical Research (ICMR). Standard Treatment Workflow (STW) for Type 2 Diabetes Mellitus, July 2022.
2. American Diabetes Association. Standards of Medical Care in Diabetes—2024. Diabetes Care.
3. Means, Casey. Good Energy: The Surprising Connection Between Metabolism and Health. 2024.
4. World Health Organization. Definition and Diagnosis of Diabetes Mellitus and Intermediate Hyperglycemia. 2006.

CHAPTER 5

CRACKING THE C-PEPTIDE CODE – WHAT IT REALLY TELLS YOU ABOUT YOUR DIABETES

C-peptide is a protein released in equal amounts with insulin from the pancreas. Unlike insulin—which can be injected—C-peptide comes only from your body's own insulin production. It helps answer a critical question:

👉 Is your pancreas still making insulin,or has it stopped?

💡 Why C-Peptide Matters – Especially in India

While international guidelines (like the ADA) recommend C-peptide testing in select or ambiguous cases, experienced Indian clinicians use it more broadly to:

- Accurately classify the type of diabetes (Type 1, Type 2, LADA, MODY)
- Assess whether insulin is truly needed
- Predict potential for diabetes remission

– Help reduce or stop insulin when the beta cell reserve is adequate

India's diabetic population is unique, with many lean individuals, early-onset cases, and misclassified patients. C-peptide is a cost-effective, underused test that can guide the right treatment.

📌 When Should You Measure C-Peptide?

Clinical Scenario	Why It's Useful
Newly diagnosed (especially < 40 years old or lean)	Helps identify the correct type of diabetes
On insulin, unsure if still needed	Can guide safe insulin withdrawal if the pancreas is still working
Considering diabetes remission	High C-peptide indicates good beta cell reserve
Unexplained hypoglycemia	Helps differentiate between self-injected vs. body-made insulin
Poorly controlled despite medication	Detects whether the pancreas is failing or if insulin resistance is dominant

⏱ Fasting vs. Post-Meal C-Peptide – Which One?

Test	Purpose
Fasting C-peptide	Measures your pancreas's baseline activity

Post-meal (2 hours after eating)	Assesses stimulated insulin response

In Indian practice, post-meal C-peptide is more commonly used, especially when evaluating potential for diabetes reversal or checking residual beta cell activity.

📊 Interpreting Your C-Peptide Levels

C-Peptide Value	What It Indicates
< 0.3 ng/mL	Severe insulin deficiency (likely Type 1 or LADA)
0.3 – 1.0 ng/mL	Low beta cell function – insulin may be required
1.1 – 2.0 ng/mL	Moderate insulin production – oral meds may work
> 2.0 ng/mL	Likely insulin resistance – avoid insulin if possible

Always interpret your C-peptide along with:

- Blood glucose levels at the time of the test
- Kidney function, as C-peptide is cleared through the kidneys

🔚 Final Word

C-peptide testing bridges the gap between just treating sugar levels and truly understanding pancreatic function.

Whether you're clarifying a diagnosis, reassessing insulin need, or exploring remission, it gives vital insights into how much help your pancreas is still offering.

It's time this powerful but simple test becomes part of routine diabetes care in India.

References

1. American Diabetes Association. Standards of Medical Care in Diabetes—2024. Diabetes Care. 2024;47(Suppl 1):S1-S300.
2. Kalra S, Sahay R, Unnikrishnan AG. Clinical Use of C-Peptide in Diabetes Care in India. J Assoc Physicians India. 2020;68(6):35-38.
3. National Institute of Nutrition, India. Diabetes and C-Peptide Testing: Position Paper. Hyderabad, 2023.
4. ADA Clinical Compendium: Differentiating Type 1 and Type 2 Diabetes Using C-peptide. 2023.

CHAPTER 6

ESSENTIAL TEST IN DIABETES – WHAT TO MEASURE, WHAT THEY MEAN?

Managing diabetes isn't just about checking blood sugar levels occasionally. It's about staying ahead of complications through regular, targeted testing. This chapter offers a practical guide to the must-do tests for people living with diabetes—what they mean, how often to do them, and how to interpret the results.

HbA1c (Glycated Hemoglobin)

- Measures average blood sugar over 2–3 months.
- Frequency: Every 3–6 months.
- Target: <7% (individualized based on age/comorbidities).
- High levels = Poor control; increases risk of complications.

Fasting Blood Sugar (FBS)

- Measures blood glucose after 8–10 hours of fasting.
- Frequency: Monthly or as advised.
- Target: 80–130 mg/dL.
- Helps in daily monitoring and treatment adjustment.

Postprandial Blood Sugar (PPBS)

- Measures sugar 2 hours after a meal.
- Frequency: Monthly or as advised.
- Target: <180 mg/dL.
- Reflects how well the body manages sugar spikes.

Continuous Glucose Monitoring (CGM)

- Tracks real-time sugar variations and trends.
- Frequency: Periodically (2–4 times a year or during uncontrolled sugars).
- Useful for adjusting diet, insulin, and activity.

Urine Microalbumin

- Detects early kidney damage.
- Frequency: Once a year (more often if positive).
- Normal: <30 mg/g creatinine.
- Early detection can prevent progression to kidney failure.

Lipid Profile

- Checks cholesterol and triglyceride levels.
- Frequency: Yearly (or 6-monthly if abnormal).

- Targets: LDL <100 mg/dL, HDL >40/50 mg/dL, Triglycerides <150 mg/dL.
- Cardiovascular risk management is essential in diabetes.

Serum Creatinine & eGFR

- Assesses kidney function.
- Frequency: Yearly (or more often if abnormal).
- eGFR >90 is normal; <60 indicates chronic kidney disease.

Liver Function Tests (LFTs)

- Screens for fatty liver and liver damage.
- Frequency: Yearly.
- Elevated ALT, AST may suggest NAFLD (common in diabetes).

Thyroid Profile (TSH, T3, T4)

- Hypothyroidism can worsen sugar control.
- Frequency: Yearly or if symptoms arise.
- Abnormal levels may need endocrinologist review.

Vitamin B12 and Vitamin D

- Metformin can lower B12; D deficiency is common in India.
- Frequency: Yearly.
- Supplement if levels are low.

Eye (Fundus) Examination

- Detects diabetic retinopathy.
- Frequency: Yearly.

- Essential even in asymptomatic patients.

Foot Exam (Neuropathy Screening)

- Checks sensation, circulation, and foot ulcers.
- Frequency: Yearly (or more for high-risk patients).
- Prevents serious complications like amputations.

Blood Pressure Monitoring

- Hypertension worsens diabetic complications.
- Frequency: Every visit.
- Target: <130/80 mmHg.

ECG / Cardiac Screening

- Detects silent heart disease.
- Frequency: Yearly or based on symptoms/risk.
- Diabetes is equivalent to heart disease risk.

Ultrasound Abdomen (USG)

- Helps detect fatty liver (NAFLD), which is common in diabetics.
- Frequency: Once during initial diagnosis and as advised.
- Fatty liver contributes to insulin resistance and increases diabetes complications.

High-Sensitivity C-Reactive Protein (hs-CRP)

- Marker of low-grade inflammation and cardiovascular risk.
- Frequency: Once a year or as advised.

- High levels indicate increased heart disease risk even if sugars are under control.

Homocysteine

- Elevated levels are linked to cardiovascular disease and nerve damage.
- Frequency: Periodically, especially in high-risk individuals.
- Controlled through B-vitamin supplementation if high.

Quick Recap

Here's a simplified overview of the essential tests every person with diabetes should track periodically:

Test Name	Frequency	Why It Matters
HbA1c	Every 3–6 months	Average glucose control over 3 months
Fasting Blood Sugar	Monthly	Daily sugar management
Postprandial Blood Sugar	Monthly	Glucose spike management
CGM	Quarterly (if needed)	Real-time sugar insights
Urine Microalbumin	Yearly	Early kidney damage detection
Lipid Profile	Yearly	Heart disease risk
Creatinine/eGFR	Yearly	Kidney function

Liver Function Tests	Yearly	Fatty liver assessment
Thyroid Profile	Yearly	Sugar-hormone balance
Vitamin B12 & D	Yearly	Prevent deficiency-related issues
Eye Exam (Fundus)	Yearly	Detects diabetic retinopathy
Foot Exam	Yearly	Neuropathy & ulcer prevention
Blood Pressure	Every visit	Heart and kidney protection
ECG/Cardiac Screening	Yearly	Detect silent heart problems
USG Abdomen	At diagnosis, then as advised	Fatty liver detection
hs-CRP	Yearly	Inflammation and cardiac risk
Homocysteine	Yearly	Cardiac and nerve health

References

1. American Diabetes Association. Standards of Medical Care in Diabetes—2025. Diabetes Care. 2025.
2. International Diabetes Federation (IDF) Clinical Practice Recommendations. 2023.

3. Diabetes Prevention Program (DPP) Study Group. NEJM. 2002.
4. National Kidney Foundation Guidelines on Chronic Kidney Disease. 2023.
5. UK Prospective Diabetes Study (UKPDS). Lancet. 1998.
6. DiRECT Trial. Lean MEJ, et al. Lancet. 2018.
7. Indian Council of Medical Research (ICMR) Guidelines for Diabetes Management. 2023.

CHAPTER 7

I FEEL FINE... SO WHY WORRY? THE SILENT DAMAGE OF HIGH BLOOD SUGAR

Many people with high blood sugar levels believe that if they feel okay, there's no cause for concern. Unfortunately, Type 2 diabetes often works silently, damaging the body long before symptoms arise. This false sense of security can lead to devastating consequences if proactive steps aren't taken early.

What Happens Inside While You Feel 'Fine'

Even when you don't experience symptoms, elevated blood sugar starts to damage small and large blood vessels, nerve endings, and vital organs. Glycation — a process where sugar attaches to proteins — disrupts normal cellular function, leading to oxidative stress and inflammation. Over time, this silent assault lays the foundation for long-term complications.

The Timeline of Silent Damage

- 1–3 years: Microvascular damage begins in the kidneys, eyes, and nerves.
- 5+ years: Early signs of complications like retinopathy, neuropathy, and sexual dysfunction emerge.
- 10+ years: Risk of stroke, heart disease, chronic kidney disease, and amputations increases, often before any warning signs.

Major Complications to Watch For

- Diabetic Retinopathy – Damage to the small vessels in the eyes, leading to vision loss.
- Diabetic Nephropathy – Kidney damage that begins silently and can progress to kidney failure.
- Diabetic Neuropathy – Nerve damage that causes tingling, numbness, and foot ulcers.
- Cardiovascular Disease – Heart attacks and strokes occur more frequently in diabetics.
- Foot Complications – Poor healing due to nerve and vessel damage can lead to amputation.
- Erectile Dysfunction – A common but often ignored early sign of vascular damage in men.

What Tests Reveal (Even When You Feel Normal)

Routine tests such as HbA1c, fasting and post-meal blood glucose, urine microalbumin, retinal scans, and foot exams can detect early damage. Continuous Glucose Monitoring (CGM) can help identify sugar spikes you may never feel, offering a clear picture of your real-time glucose control.

The Power of Prevention

Controlling blood sugar levels early can drastically reduce the risk of complications. According to global data, tight control within the first five years can cut the risk of long-term complications by 70%. Even modest improvements in lifestyle can lead to major metabolic health gains.

Key Takeaways

- You can feel fine and still be on the path to serious diabetes complications.
- Silent damage affects your eyes, kidneys, nerves, heart, and sexual health.
- Early testing and tight control prevent or reverse complications.
- The best time to act is before symptoms appear—not after.

References

1. American Diabetes Association. Standards of Medical Care in Diabetes—2025. Diabetes Care. 2025;48(Supplement_1):S1–S212.
2. UK Prospective Diabetes Study (UKPDS). Intensive blood-glucose control with sulphonylureas or insulin compared with conventional treatment. Lancet. 1998.
3. DiRECT Trial. Lean MEJ, et al. Lancet. 2018;391(10120):541–551.
4. Diabetes Prevention Program (DPP) Research Group. Reduction in the incidence of type 2 diabetes with lifestyle intervention. NEJM. 2002.

5. Saenz A, et al. Metformin monotherapy for type 2 diabetes mellitus. Cochrane Database Syst Rev. 2005.
6. Tesfaye S, et al. Diabetic neuropathies: update on definitions, diagnostic criteria, estimation of severity, and treatments. Diabetes Care. 2010.
7. International Diabetes Federation (IDF) Clinical Practice Recommendations for Managing Type 2 Diabetes in Primary Care. 2023.

CHAPTER 8

DIABETES AT 30? WHY YOUNG INDIANS ARE CRASHING EARLY AND HOW TO CHANGE COURSE

Type 2 diabetes was once called 'adult-onset' for a reason. But not anymore. In India, a rising number of individuals between the ages of 25 and 35 are being diagnosed with Type 2 diabetes, often without warning. This chapter explores the reasons behind this alarming trend, its long-term consequences, and what can be done to prevent or reverse it.

👥 The New Face of Diabetes in India

- India is witnessing a silent epidemic of early-onset Type 2 diabetes, with cases being reported in people as young as 18.
- Factors include increased fast-food consumption, late-night eating, sedentary digital lifestyles, and high levels of stress.

– Many of these young patients are non-obese and unaware of their metabolic dysfunction.

🔍 Why Are 25-Year-Olds Getting Type 2 Diabetes?

– Genetics: Indians have a stronger genetic predisposition to insulin resistance (the 'thin-fat' Indian phenotype).
– Diet: High refined carbohydrate intake (maida, sugary beverages) from childhood.
– PCOS in women and fatty liver in men often go unnoticed until sugars spike.
– Sleep deprivation and excessive screen time reduce insulin sensitivity.

⚠ Early Diabetes = Early Complications

Getting diabetes in your 20s or 30s gives the disease decades to cause damage. Studies show:

– Early-onset diabetes is linked with faster progression of complications like retinopathy, kidney disease, and heart failure.
– Many are undiagnosed until a major event—vision problems, stroke, infertility—forces a check-up.
– Long-term exposure to high glucose means longer cumulative damage.

🔄 Can Young-Onset Diabetes Be Reversed?

Yes—in many cases. Because younger bodies are more metabolically flexible, lifestyle changes often lead to rapid improvements. Sustainable reversal is possible through:

- Low-carb, protein-rich diets with mindful portion control
- Intermittent fasting or circadian eating
- Physical activity: 45+ minutes of brisk walking, HIIT, or strength training
- Quality sleep and stress reduction
- Periodic follow-ups with a proactive physician

A Wake-Up Call for Young India

Type 2 diabetes isn't just a lifestyle disease—it's a life-course disease. The earlier it starts, the more serious it becomes. But this generation also has tools that the previous ones didn't: better diagnostics, food awareness, wearables, and social support. Take control early, and you might never have to suffer the full burden of the disease.

Quick Recap

- An increasing number of Indians are being diagnosed with Type 2 diabetes between the ages of 25–35.
- Early-onset diabetes is linked to modern sedentary lifestyles, processed diets, and sleep disruption.
- Genetics, PCOS, and fatty liver play major roles—even in those who appear lean.
- This form of diabetes tends to progress faster and carries a higher risk of complications.
- Early intervention through diet, exercise, and metabolic monitoring can reverse or control the disease.

References

1. Anjana RM, et al. Younger-onset Type 2 Diabetes and its Impact. Diabetologia. 2023;66(4):567–578.
2. Mohan V, et al. Epidemiology of Type 2 Diabetes in India. Indian J Med Res. 2022;155(4):387–395.
3. IDF Diabetes Atlas, 11th Edition. International Diabetes Federation, 2024.
4. Kaur P, et al. Early-onset Type 2 Diabetes: Risk Factors and Clinical Profile. J Assoc Physicians India. 2023;71(5):25–31.
5. Nanditha A, et al. The rising burden of diabetes and youth in India. Lancet Diabetes Endocrinol. 2024;12(2):109–117.

CHAPTER 9

DIABETES IN WOMEN – UNSEEN, UNEQUAL, UNSPOKEN

Introduction

Diabetes doesn't affect everyone the same way. In women, it hides behind hormonal shifts, cultural silence, and often delayed diagnosis. From puberty to menopause, a woman's journey with diabetes is uniquely complex, and dangerously under-acknowledged.

1. The Female Hormonal Terrain: A Diabetic Minefield

Women's hormones modulate insulin sensitivity, fat distribution, and even appetite.

- Estrogen and progesterone fluctuations influence glucose metabolism.
- Blood sugar control often worsens during PMS, menopause transition, and PCOS.
- These are metabolic accelerants.

2. PCOS: The Early Warning

Polycystic Ovary Syndrome (PCOS) is an insulin-resistant state, often a precursor to Type 2 diabetes.

- 70% of the women with PCOS have insulin resistance.
- Often mismanaged for cosmetic concerns.
- Early lifestyle intervention can delay diabetes.

3. Menopause: The Unmasked Metabolic Storm

Estrogen decline leads to visceral fat and insulin resistance.

- Symptoms overlap with menopause: fatigue, hot flashes, sleep issues.
- Cardiometabolic risk rises.
- Midlife screening is essential.

4. The Cardiovascular Time Bomb

Women with diabetes are 3–7x more likely to die from heart disease.

- Atypical symptoms lead to underdiagnosis.
- Markers like ApoB, Lp(a), hs-CRP should be screened.

5. Mental Load & Emotional Burnout

Women often delay care due to family priorities.

- Emotional eating, depression are common.
- Stigma around reproductive health leads to neglect.

6. Societal Blind Spots

In India, testing often happens only after complications.

- Pregnancy and menopause remain under-screened metabolic windows.
- Diabetes is often seen as a male problem, which it is not.

Quick Recap

- PCOS is metabolic.
- Menopause worsens metabolic risk.
- Heart disease risk is greater in diabetic women.
- Emotional health is equally critical.

What Every Woman Must Ask Her Doctor — A Life Stage Guide

Life Stage	– Key Screenings & Questions
Adolescence / PCOS	– Fasting insulin, HOMA-IR, OGTT – Pelvic ultrasound – Ask: "Am I insulin resistant?"
Reproductive Age (20s–30s)	– Fasting glucose, HbA1c – Menstrual history – Ask: "Am I at risk of future diabetes?"
Preconception Planning	– HbA1c (<6.5%) – Thyroid panel, Vitamin D – Ask: "Is my sugar safe for pregnancy?"

Postpartum (GDM history)	– OGTT 6–12 weeks post-delivery – Annual metabolic screening – Ask: "How do I prevent Type 2 diabetes?"
Perimenopause (40s–50s)	– Lipids (ApoB, Lp(a)) – HbA1c, OGTT – Ask: "Is menopause affecting my sugar and heart?"
Postmenopause	– DEXA scan – hs-CRP, HOMA-IR – Ask: "Am I protected from heart disease and fractures?"
Any Age (with risk)	– Annual HbA1c & insulin check – Lifestyle counselling

References

1. Legro RS, et al. Diagnosis and treatment of PCOS: An Endocrine Society Clinical Practice Guideline. J Clin Endocrinol Metab. 2013.
2. Wild S, et al. Cardiovascular disease in women with diabetes. BMJ. 2007.
3. Pinkhasov RM, et al. Gender differences in the quality of care among diabetic patients. Diabetes Care. 2008.
4. Indian Menopause Society: Clinical Practice Guidelines 2022.
5. RSSDI 2023 Position Statement on Diabetes in Women.

CHAPTER 10

SKINNY BUT SICK – INDIA'S HIDDEN DIABETICS

Introduction

"But I'm not fat… how can I have diabetes?"

This is a question doctors hear every day, especially in India. For decades, we've equated diabetes with obesity. But research now reveals a startling truth: you can look slim and still be metabolically unhealthy. Welcome to the world of TOFI—Thin Outside, Fat Inside.

The TOFI Phenotype: A Silent Danger

TOFI refers to individuals who have a normal BMI but excess visceral fat—fat wrapped around internal organs like the liver, pancreas, and intestines. This fat is metabolically active and strongly linked to:

- Insulin resistance
- Fatty liver (NAFLD)

– Inflammation
– Type 2 diabetes
– Cardiovascular disease

Why India Is Ground Zero for TOFI

South Asians, particularly Indians, are genetically and environmentally predisposed to this hidden fat accumulation:

– We develop insulin resistance at lower BMI levels than Caucasians.
– Our body fat is preferentially stored viscerally, not subcutaneously.
– We often have lower muscle mass (sarcopenia) with poor physical activity levels.
– Cultural diets often include refined carbs, sweets, and trans fats with minimal protein or fiber.

The "Normal BMI" Trap

BMI is a poor indicator of metabolic health in Indians. Many diabetics are missed in the early stages because:

– Their weight is "normal"
– They feel fine
– Their fasting sugar might still be in the high-normal range

But if tested, these individuals may have:

– High fasting insulin
– High triglycerides
– Fatty liver on ultrasound
– Acanthosis nigricans (dark neck folds)

The Right Tests: Going Beyond Blood Sugar

To detect TOFI or early insulin resistance in slim individuals, the following tests are more revealing:

- HOMA-IR
- Fasting insulin levels
- Triglyceride/HDL ratio
- Liver function tests
- Waist circumference
- DEXA scan or MRI fat mapping

What Causes Slim Diabetics?

Even without obesity, a deadly combination of urban stress, poor sleep, processed food, low protein intake, and inactivity creates the perfect storm:

- Late-night meals + screen exposure
- Skipping breakfast or eating carb-heavy meals
- Muscle loss (sarcopenia) with age or low protein intake

Case Study: A 32-Year-Old Banker With Diabetes

Ravi was 32, weighed 65 kg, BMI 22. He looked "fit." But chronic fatigue, belly bloating, and darkening of the neck led to a health check:

- Fasting insulin: 21 μIU/mL
- HOMA-IR: 5.1
- HbA1c: 6.6%
- Fatty liver on ultrasound

Ravi was a TOFI. With lifestyle intervention and intermittent fasting, he reversed his markers in 6 months, without medications.

The Good News: It's Reversible

The TOFI condition is fully reversible if caught early. Key interventions include:

- Time-restricted eating (16:8 IF)
- Strength training
- High-protein diet
- Cutting refined carbs
- Sleep hygiene and stress management

Why This Matters: The Invisible Epidemic

India is facing an epidemic not just of diabetes, but of "invisible diabetics." TOFI individuals often:

- Get diagnosed late
- Face complications earlier
- Feel confused because they never "looked sick"

Key Signs You Might Be a TOFI

- Slim but have belly fat
- Tired after meals
- Frequent cravings
- Borderline sugar but high insulin
- Fatty liver or PCOS with normal weight

References

1. Mohan V, et al. Diabetes Technology & Therapeutics, 2010.
2. Thomas EL, et al. Obesity Reviews, 2012.
3. Misra A, et al. Journal of Diabetes Science and Technology, 2011.
4. NDTV.com, 2023.
5. WHO South-East Asia report, 2021.

CHAPTER 11

THE INFLAMMATION EQUATION – WHY DIABETES ISN'T JUST ABOUT SUGAR

> "If you only chase sugar, you'll miss the fire."

Beyond Blood Sugar – The Hidden Inflammation Driving Diabetes

For years, diabetes has been treated as a sugar problem. But emerging science paints a different picture: chronic low-grade inflammation begins long before glucose rises, and it continues silently, damaging blood vessels, insulin receptors, and organs even when blood sugars are "under control."

This silent, systemic inflammation, also known as metaflammation, is measurable, reversible, and often overlooked.

What Is Chronic Low-Grade Inflammation?

Unlike acute inflammation (which helps us heal from injury or infection), chronic inflammation is subtle and persistent. It's driven by dysfunctional fat cells, gut-derived toxins, poor sleep, stress, and processed food—and it disrupts the body's ability to use insulin properly.

This internal "fire" keeps insulin levels elevated, blocks fat loss, and damages pancreatic beta cells over time, setting the stage for type 2 diabetes and its complications.

Inflammation Markers That Reveal the Metabolic Fire

These blood-based biomarkers are now recognized as critical in understanding the metabolic state beyond glucose:

Marker	Ideal Range	Why It Matters
hs-CRP	<1 mg/L	A general marker of systemic inflammation; values >3 mg/L are strongly linked to heart disease in diabetics
IL-6	<1.5 pg/mL	A cytokine from visceral fat and immune cells; promotes liver glucose output and worsens insulin resistance
TNF-α	<5 pg/mL	Suppresses insulin signaling, promotes fat inflammation and beta-cell damage

MCP-1	—	Recruits immune cells into fat tissue; not yet routine but rising in research use
Fibrinogen	200–400 mg/dL	An inflammatory clotting factor; high levels increase cardiovascular risk in diabetes
Ferritin	<100 ng/mL	Acts as an acute-phase reactant; elevated in inflammation even with normal iron stores
Adiponectin	>6 µg/mL	A protective, anti-inflammatory hormone; levels drop in insulin resistance and TOFI (thin outside, fat inside) individuals

How Inflammation Disrupts Glucose Metabolism

- Cytokines like IL-6 and TNF-α block insulin signaling pathways inside cells.
- They increase hepatic gluconeogenesis (sugar production in the liver).
- They cause beta-cell apoptosis, reducing insulin secretion over time.
- They elevate vascular risk, even when blood sugar and cholesterol seem "normal."

Yearly Preventive Testing – What to Measure and Why

For individuals with diabetes, prediabetes, or central obesity, these inflammatory markers should be included in annual metabolic screening:

Strongly Recommended Annually:

Marker	Use	Ideal Range
hs-CRP	Predicts vascular risk, reflects systemic inflammation	<1 mg/L
Fibrinogen	Indicates clotting and inflammation	200–400 mg/dL
Ferritin	Signals low-grade inflammation	<100 ng/mL (in non-anemic patients)

Consider in High-Risk or Resistant Cases:

Marker	Use	Suggested Frequency	Ideal Range
IL-6	In unexplained insulin resistance or TOFI phenotype	Every 1–2 years	<1.5 pg/mL

TNF-α	Persistent fatigue, inflammation despite normal HbA1c	1–2 years	<5 pg/mL
Adiponectin	In lean diabetics or metabolic syndrome with normal BMI	Once or if needed	>6 μg/mL

What Lowers Inflammation (And Improves Glucose Too)

Food as Medicine:

- Emphasize: Turmeric, omega-3s (fish/flax), extra virgin olive oil, berries, green leafy vegetables, fermented foods
- Avoid: Sugar, refined flours, seed oils (sunflower, soybean), fried snacks

Movement:

- Brisk walking + resistance training lowers TNF-α and increases adiponectin

Sleep & Stress:

- Just 1 night of poor sleep raises IL-6 and CRP
- Yoga, mindfulness, pranayama reduce cortisol and sympathetic overdrive

Medications:

- Metformin – mild anti-inflammatory effects on the liver and gut
- SGLT2 inhibitors & GLP-1 agonists – reduce inflammation and cardiovascular risk
- Omega-3 supplements (EPA/DHA) – reduce IL-6 and CRP

Conclusion: Track the Fire, Not Just the Flame

"Sugar is the symptom. Inflammation is the cause."

You can't manage diabetes effectively without recognizing and addressing chronic inflammation.

Routine blood sugar tests are important, but they're not enough. A yearly inflammation profile, even as simple as hs-CRP and ferritin, can reveal the true metabolic status.

The earlier you detect and cool the internal fire, the more you can prevent complications—and possibly, reverse the course of disease.

References

1. Donath MY, Shoelson SE. Type 2 diabetes as an inflammatory disease. Nat Rev Immunol. 2011 Feb;11(2):98–107.
2. Pradhan AD, Manson JE, Rifai N, Buring JE, Ridker PM. C-reactive protein, interleukin 6, and risk of developing type 2 diabetes mellitus. JAMA. 2001 Jul 18;286(3):327–34.
3. Hotamisligil GS. Inflammation and metabolic disorders. Nature. 2006 Dec 14;444(7121):860–7.

4. Pickup JC. Inflammation and activated innate immunity in the pathogenesis of type 2 diabetes. Diabetes Care. 2004 Mar;27(3):813–23.
5. Kolb H, Mandrup-Poulsen T. The global diabetes epidemic as a consequence of lifestyle-induced low-grade inflammation. Diabetologia. 2010 Jan;53(1):10–20.
6. Ridker PM et al. C-reactive protein and other markers of inflammation in the prediction of cardiovascular disease in women. N Engl J Med. 2000 Mar 23;342(12):836–43.
7. Chawla A, Nguyen KD, Goh YP. Macrophage-mediated inflammation in metabolic disease. Nat Rev Immunol. 2011 Nov;11(11):738–49.
8. Wellen KE, Hotamisligil GS. Inflammation, stress, and diabetes. J Clin Invest. 2005 May;115(5):1111–9.
9. Esser N, Legrand-Poels S, Piette J, Scheen AJ, Paquot N. Inflammation as a link between obesity, metabolic syndrome and type 2 diabetes. Diabetes Res Clin Pract. 2014 Aug;105(2):141–50.

CHAPTER 12

TOXIC BLOOD SUGAR – HOW EVERYDAY CHEMICALS DISRUPT METABOLISM AND CAUSE DIABETES

Over the past few decades, the rates of Type 2 Diabetes have skyrocketed — not just due to poor diet or lack of exercise, but because of a lesser-known factor: exposure to everyday environmental toxins. These include plastics, pesticides, air pollutants, and household chemicals that silently disrupt metabolic health.

🔬 What Are Endocrine-Disrupting Chemicals (EDCs)?

EDCs are substances that interfere with hormonal systems in the body. They mimic, block, or alter hormones, particularly insulin, leading to insulin resistance, increased fat storage, and inflammation — all of which contribute to the development of diabetes.

🧴 Common Metabolic Disruptors and Where They Hide

- BPA (Bisphenol A): Found in plastic bottles, food containers, and linings of canned foods.
- Phthalates: Present in cosmetics, perfumes, plastic wraps, and vinyl flooring.
- Pesticides: Residues on fruits and vegetables, especially non-organic produce.
- Heavy Metals: Such as arsenic and cadmium in groundwater or industrial areas.
- Air Pollutants: From vehicle exhaust, industrial emissions, and indoor cooking fumes.

📚 Scientific Evidence Linking EDCs to Diabetes

Numerous studies have found associations between EDC exposure and Type 2 Diabetes. For instance:

- A 2022 review in *The Lancet Diabetes & Endocrinology* concluded that BPA exposure is positively linked with insulin resistance.
- Indian studies have reported higher diabetes risk in people living near industrial or heavily polluted areas.
- Research from the National Institutes of Health (NIH) supports the role of phthalates and other EDCs in disrupting pancreatic beta-cell function.

🛡 How to Reduce Your Exposure – Indian Lifestyle Tips

- Use stainless steel or glass containers instead of plastic for food storage.
- Wash fruits and vegetables thoroughly; consider peeling if not organic.
- Choose cosmetics and personal care products labeled 'phthalate-free' and 'paraben-free'.
- Avoid heating food in plastic containers, especially in microwaves.
- Use exhaust fans or proper ventilation while cooking indoors.
- Filter drinking water if living in areas with known contamination risks.

🌍 The Bigger Picture – Diabetes Beyond Diet

Understanding the environmental contributors to diabetes shifts the focus from just personal choices to societal and policy-level interventions. It also helps explain why even non-obese individuals or those eating reasonably well might still develop diabetes—it's not just about calories anymore.

🔁 Quick Recap

- Endocrine-disrupting chemicals (EDCs) are hidden in plastics, cosmetics, pesticides, and even air.
- These chemicals can interfere with insulin action, promote fat storage, and raise diabetes risk.
- Common EDCs include BPA, phthalates, and pesticide residues in food and water.

- Scientific studies strongly link EDC exposure to increased risk of Type 2 Diabetes.
- Simple lifestyle changes like using glass containers, avoiding plastic reheating, and filtering water can help reduce exposure.

📚 References

1. Heindel JJ, et al. Endocrine-disrupting chemicals and risk of diabetes. Lancet Diabetes Endocrinol. 2022;10(3):189–205.
2. Rajesh P, et al. Urban pollution and the rising prevalence of diabetes in Indian cities. J Diabetol. 2023;14(2):54–60.
3. National Institute of Environmental Health Sciences (NIEHS). Endocrine Disruptors and Metabolic Disorders. NIH Report, 2024.
4. Trasande L, et al. Phthalates and Metabolic Dysfunction: Current Evidence and Public Health Implications. Rev Endocr Metab Disord. 2021;22(2):241–256.
5. Indian Council of Medical Research. Environmental Risk Factors for Non-Communicable Diseases. ICMR Report, 2023.

CHAPTER 13

DIGITAL DIABETES – HOW SCREENS, SLEEP LOSS, AND SOCIAL MEDIA ARE SPIKING YOUR SUGARS

Introduction

In a hyperconnected world, we scroll more than we sleep, and binge-watch more than we breathe deeply. This digital overload is silently driving up stress, disturbing sleep, and worsening blood sugar control. This chapter reveals how screen addiction is contributing to the diabetes epidemic—and how to regain metabolic balance without giving up modern life.

1. Blue Light at Night – The Sleep Destroyer

– Screens emit blue light that suppresses melatonin, delaying deep sleep.

- Poor sleep impairs glucose metabolism, increases cortisol, and raises next-day blood sugar.
- Studies show just 5 nights of poor sleep can reduce insulin sensitivity by 20–25%.

2. Social Media = Cortisol Spikes + Sugar Cravings

- Doomscrolling, comparison, and emotional triggers raise cortisol.
- High cortisol increases abdominal fat and blood glucose.
- The dopamine hits from reels, likes, and comments keep us addicted—and more likely to snack impulsively.

3. Sedentary Tech Time = Glucose Buildup

- Hours of sitting with gadgets = reduced muscle activity = reduced glucose disposal.
- Insulin needs movement to work effectively—every 30 minutes of sitting should be broken by standing or walking.
- Even small actions like standing phone calls or post-reel stretches help.

4. Screen Time and Kids – Sowing Seeds of Early Diabetes

- Children glued to screens snack more, move less, and sleep worse.
- Increasing evidence links screen time to childhood obesity and early insulin resistance.
- Parents should model healthy tech behavior.

5. Sleep Hygiene – Reset Your Tech-Life Balance

✅ Practical Fixes:

- No screens 1 hour before bed
- Use night mode or blue light filters in the evening
- Read physical books, journal, or meditate before sleeping
- Keep phones out of the bedroom if possible
- Fixed sleep-wake time trains the circadian rhythm

6. Build a Digital Diet for Diabetes Health

- Set time limits on apps
- Use a real alarm clock (avoid waking to notifications)
- Use screen time reports to reduce unconscious usage
- Use apps that track habits, movement, and hydration instead of only consuming content

7. Tech That Helps, Not Hurts

✅ Use tech tools that support glucose control:

- CGMs (Continuous Glucose Monitors)
- Fitness trackers
- Mindfulness apps (Headspace, Insight Timer)
- YouTube channels with guided workouts or yoga

Tech is not the enemy—it's how we use it.

Success Story: Rahul, 28 – Gamer to Glucose-Aware

Rahul, a techie and gamer, had borderline diabetes and triglycerides of 360. He:

- Cut screen time after 9 PM

– Took 10-minute walks after meals while listening to audiobooks
– Switched from late-night gaming to early morning walking

His HbA1c dropped from 6.1% to 5.6% in 4 months, with no meds.

Takeaway

You don't need to go offline. You need to go intentional.

Reclaim your attention, protect your sleep, and move your body—even in a digital world.

"The more conscious your screen use, the more stable your sugars."

References

1. Spiegel K, Leproult R, Van Cauter E. Impact of sleep debt on metabolic and endocrine function. The Lancet. 1999;354(9188):1435–1439.
2. Buxton OM, Pavlova M, Reid EW, Wang W, Simonson DC, Adler GK. Sleep restriction for 1 week reduces insulin sensitivity in healthy men. Diabetes. 2010;59(9):2126–2133.
3. Khandelwal D, et al. Digital screen time during COVID-19 pandemic: a public health concern. Diabetes & Metabolic Syndrome: Clinical Research & Reviews. 2021;15(1):341–343.
4. Shochat T, et al. The impact of smartphone use on sleep and cognitive functioning in young adults. J Clin Sleep Med. 2020;16(10):1735–1742.

5. Taheri S, Lin L, Austin D, Young T, Mignot E. Short sleep duration is associated with reduced leptin, elevated ghrelin, and increased body mass index. PLoS Med. 2004;1(3):e62.
6. Wang Y, Lobstein T. Worldwide trends in childhood overweight and obesity. Int J Pediatr Obes. 2006;1(1):11–25.
7. Dutil C, Chaput JP. Inadequate sleep as a contributor to type 2 diabetes in children and adolescents. Nutr Diabetes. 2017;7(5):e266.
8. Gupta R, et al. Sleep disorders in the Indian population: results from a cross-sectional survey. PLoS One. 2020;15(12):e0243823.

SECTION 2

CHAPTER 1

THE TURNING POINT – CAN DIABETES GO INTO REMISSION?

Remission vs. Reversal – What's the Right Term?

The term "reversal" is often used casually, but the more accurate and medically accepted term is "remission." According to the American Diabetes Association and international consensus guidelines, diabetes remission is defined as:

- HbA1c <6.5% for at least 3 months
- Without the use of glucose-lowering medications

Remission is most achievable in people with type 2 diabetes or prediabetes. It is not typically possible in type 1 diabetes or advanced beta-cell failure cases.

The Science Behind Remission

The root of type 2 diabetes lies in excess fat, particularly in the liver and pancreas. This fat interferes with insulin action (causing resistance) and insulin secretion (beta-cell dysfunction).

The Twin Cycle Hypothesis by Professor Roy Taylor explains how reducing intra-organ fat through weight loss and lifestyle change can restore metabolic health and induce remission.

Global Evidence That Remission Is Real

Several major studies confirm that remission of type 2 diabetes is possible:

- "DiRECT Trial (UK):" Nearly 46% of participants achieved remission at 12 months using a structured low-calorie program.
- "Virta Health Study (USA):" Over 60% achieved remission with a ketogenic diet approach.
- "Indian Case Series:" Clinicians report high remission rates using lifestyle tools like low-carb diets, intermittent fasting, and yoga.

These findings suggest that remission is not just a theory—it is happening every day in clinics worldwide.

How Remission Happens – Practical Tools That Work

There is no magic pill for remission—it is the result of consistent and strategic lifestyle intervention. The most effective tools include:

- "Low-Carb or Real-Food Diets": Reduce glucose load, lower insulin demand.
- "Intermittent Fasting": Gives the pancreas rest, reduces insulin levels.
- "Strength Training & Daily Activity": Improves glucose uptake and muscle insulin sensitivity.

- "Stress Management": Cortisol control is crucial in insulin resistance.
- "Quality Sleep": Poor sleep alone can spike insulin resistance.

Doctor's Take

Over the past several years, I've guided more than 100 patients toward diabetes remission, many of whom were on multiple medications, including insulin. With a personalized approach focusing on nutrition, fasting, physical activity, and mindset, they achieved normal blood sugars without lifelong drugs. With the right guidance, remission is not just possible—it is predictable.

Timing Matters – When Is Remission Most Likely?

The earlier the intervention, the higher the chance of remission. Best outcomes are seen in:

- People with diabetes duration less than 6–8 years
- Individuals with significant visceral fat or fatty liver
- Motivated patients able to sustain lifestyle change

Remission becomes more difficult (but not impossible) after 10–15 years of diabetes, or in patients with significant beta-cell failure.

Quick Recap

- Remission (not cure) is the appropriate term for type 2 diabetes reversal.
- It's defined as HbA1c <6.5% for at least 3 months without medications.

- Remission is achievable in prediabetes and early-to-mid-stage type 2 diabetes.
- Reducing liver and pancreatic fat through diet and fasting is key.
- The earlier you act, the more likely you are to achieve long-term remission.

References

1. American Diabetes Association. Standards of Medical Care in Diabetes—2024. Diabetes Care.
2. Taylor R. The Twin Cycle Hypothesis for Type 2 Diabetes: UK DiRECT Study. The Lancet, 2018.
3. Hallberg SJ et al. Effectiveness and Safety of a Novel Care Model for the Management of Type 2 Diabetes. Virta Health Study.
4. Indian Council of Medical Research (ICMR). STW for Type 2 Diabetes Mellitus, 2022.

CHAPTER 2

THE REVERSAL CODE – HOW EARLY DIABETES CAN BE UNDONE WITHOUT MEDICATIONS

Introduction

"What if diabetes isn't a life sentence—but a warning signal you can switch off?"

Type 2 diabetes—long believed to be a progressive, lifelong condition—is now proven to be reversible, especially when caught early. And the most powerful tools aren't pills—they're lifestyle interventions.

Reversal Is Not a Myth – It's Measured Remission

Remission means your blood sugar levels return to normal or prediabetic range without medications, for at least 3 to 6 months.

- HbA1c <6.5% without medication
- Fasting glucose <100 mg/dL

– Post-meal sugar <140 mg/dL

Why Reversal Is Possible: Understanding the Root Cause

Type 2 diabetes is primarily caused by insulin resistance, not a lack of insulin. Most early-stage patients have too much insulin. The key is to reduce insulin demand and improve sensitivity by reducing organ fat and reversing metabolic dysfunction.

Global Evidence: What the Science Says

The DiRECT Trial (UK): Low-calorie diet led to 46% remission at 1 year, and 86% in those losing >15 kg.

Virta Health (USA): Low-carb approach with coaching led to 60% off meds and improved HbA1c over 2+ years.

India: Intermittent fasting, low-carb diets, yoga, and lifestyle protocols have shown high reversal rates in early diabetics.

Top Reversal Strategies – What Actually Works

– Intermittent Fasting (e.g., 16:8)
– Low-Carbohydrate or Ketogenic Diet
– Weight Loss (especially visceral fat)
– Muscle Building Exercise
– Sleep and Stress Optimization

Who Can Reverse Diabetes?

Most likely candidates include:

– Recent diagnosis (within 3–5 years)
– On oral medications only

– Residual insulin production (C-peptide positive)
– Committed to lifestyle change

Not for Everyone – But Worth Trying

Reversal may not be possible for long-standing diabetics or those with pancreatic burnout, but everyone can improve metabolic health and reduce complications.

Key Reminders for Safe Reversal

– Reduce medications under medical supervision
– Monitor sugars regularly
– Risk of hypoglycemia during fasting
– Track HbA1c, insulin, and weight changes

Success Stories from Satva Specialty Clinic

Mr. Suresh, 41 – Reversed Diabetes in 6 Months Without Medications

Corporate executive with HbA1c 7.8%. Used IF + low-carb high-protein Indian diet. HbA1c dropped to 5.9%. Fatty liver resolved. Off medications.

Mrs. Revathi, 56 – From 3 Drugs to None

On metformin, glimepiride, and statins. Followed a guided lifestyle plan including low-GI foods, resistance bands, and fasting. HbA1c dropped from 8.2% to 6.1% in 8 months. Off all meds.

Rahul, 28 – "I'm Too Young for Diabetes"

Had borderline diabetes and high TG. Focused on digital detox, sleep, and strength training. HbA1c dropped to 5.6% in 3 months.

These are just a few of the many who have changed their health trajectory at Satva Specialty Clinic.

Beyond Numbers – The Emotional Victory

Diabetes remission isn't just about lab reports. It brings confidence, energy, freedom from fear, and control over one's health journey.

References

1. Taylor R, et al. DiRECT trial. Lancet, 2018.
2. Hallberg SJ, et al. Virta Health results, 2019.
3. ADA Standards of Care, 2022.
4. Joshi SR, et al. Indian Reversal Programs. JAPI, 2021.
5. Fung J. The Diabetes Code, 2018.

CHAPTER 3

PROVEN STRATEGIES FOR PREVENTION, REMISSION, AND GOOD METABOLIC HEALTH

Type 2 diabetes is not inevitable. Decades of research and clinical practice now prove that prevention, remission, and sustained metabolic health are achievable with the right lifestyle, mindset, and support. This chapter summarizes the most evidence-backed approaches to reverse diabetes and stay metabolically resilient.

1. Sustain a Healthy Body Weight

- Losing 5–10% of excess weight improves insulin sensitivity, lowers inflammation, and helps reduce blood glucose levels.
- Studies like DiRECT and DIADEM show that >15% weight loss can induce remission in early Type 2 diabetes.
- Focus on reducing visceral fat, especially from the liver and pancreas, rather than obsessing over the scale.

2. Adopt a Low-Carb, Optimum Protein Diet

- A low-carb approach reduces post-meal sugar spikes and insulin demands.
- Include protein sources like paneer, eggs, lentils, tofu, and fish to improve satiety and preserve lean mass.
- Avoid refined carbs such as white rice, maida-based foods, and sugary snacks.
- ADA 2025 recognizes low-carb diets as effective and safe when monitored.

3. Time-Restricted Eating / Intermittent Fasting

- Eating within a 6–10 hour daily window helps reduce insulin resistance and gives beta cells time to rest.
- This approach improves metabolic flexibility and supports natural circadian rhythms.
- Should be practiced under guidance if you're on medications that lower blood sugar.

4. Daily Physical Activity

- Exercise helps muscles absorb glucose independent of insulin.
- Aim for at least 150 minutes/week of moderate-intensity aerobic activity (like brisk walking, swimming, or cycling).
- Include strength training 2–3 times a week to improve insulin action and build metabolic reserves.
- Incorporate non-exercise movement like post-meal walks and standing breaks.

5. **Prioritize Sleep Quality**

    - Sleep is critical for hormonal balance and appetite regulation.
    - Aim for 7–8 hours of consistent, quality sleep every night.
    - Sleep deprivation raises cortisol and ghrelin, increasing insulin resistance and cravings.

6. **Manage Stress Effectively**

    - Chronic stress elevates cortisol, which disrupts glucose regulation and contributes to belly fat.
    - Daily stress management practices like deep breathing, journaling, mindfulness, or prayer can reset the nervous system.
    - Managing emotional health is foundational for long-term metabolic control.

7. **Support a Healthy Gut Microbiome**

    - Your gut bacteria influence glucose metabolism, immunity, and inflammation.
    - Eat prebiotic-rich foods like garlic, onions, bananas, and methi seeds.
    - Include probiotics like curd, buttermilk, and fermented vegetables to restore microbial diversity.

8. **Smart Monitoring and Early Detection**

    - Catch prediabetes and insulin resistance early to prevent full-blown diabetes.

- Track fasting and post-meal glucose, HbA1c, waist circumference, and weight.
- CGMs (Continuous Glucose Monitors) give real-time data to fine-tune food and activity choices.

9. Evidence-Based Supplementation

- Micronutrient deficiencies are common in diabetes and worsen insulin resistance.
- Supplements like Vitamin D, B12, Magnesium, Zinc, Omega-3, Berberine, and ALA support metabolic repair.
- Always consult a healthcare provider before starting supplements.

10. Build a Purpose-Driven Lifestyle

- People who are motivated by meaning and personal goals have better long-term health outcomes.
- Anchor your health journey to relationships, career, spirituality, or service.
- Purpose transforms discipline into devotion and prevents relapse.

11. Avoid Metabolic Disruptors

- Ultra-processed foods, sugary drinks, alcohol, smoking, and chronic screen exposure disrupt glucose metabolism.
- Minimize these to preserve insulin sensitivity, energy, and cellular health.

SECTION 3

NEW RULES OF NUTRITION FOR BLOOD SUGAR CONTROL

CHAPTER 1

BREAKING NORMS, BREAKING DIETARY MISCONCEPTIONS

In a typical 15-minute consultation, most physicians don't have the time to discuss the complexities of a diabetes-friendly diet. When I ask patients about their eating habits, the most common response I hear is: "We've stopped eating rice and only eat wheat chapatis." This reflects a widespread misconception.

⚠ The reality is: "wheat significantly raises blood sugar levels". Its glycemic index is comparable to that of white rice. Both are refined carbohydrates that cause sharp glucose and insulin spikes.

The ideal diabetes diet is one that "prevents post-meal blood sugar spikes" to levels that cause organ damage or complications.

Let's break down the impact of macronutrients:

- "Carbohydrates": Raise blood sugar and insulin the most
- "Proteins": Mildly increase blood sugar and insulin
- "Fats": Least impact on both sugar and insulin

Sustained intake of high-carbohydrate diets forces the pancreas to secrete more insulin, leading to hyperinsulinemia and insulin resistance, major drivers of inflammation and metabolic dysfunction.

Among carbohydrates, refined types—"maida, bread, pasta, white rice, and even wheat flour"—are the most harmful.

☑ The best dietary approach for diabetes is a "real food, low-carbohydrate diet", which includes:

- "Natural fats": coconut, coconut oil, ghee, butter, paneer, olives, nuts, seeds
- "Moderate protein": "At least 1 gram per kg body weight/day"; best sources include "eggs, paneer, Greek yogurt, fish, and chicken"
- "Non-starchy vegetables": spinach, gourds, methi, cauliflower, cucumber

Despite years of 'low-fat' dietary advice, modern research proves that "natural fats do not increase weight or LDL cholesterol" the way processed trans fats do.

📊 From "2017 to 2025", over "100 of my patients have experienced diabetes remission" by embracing a structured, low-carb, real food approach.

Books like "Good Energy by Dr. Casey Means" and peer-reviewed journals such as *The BMJ* and *Diabetes Therapy* validate this approach. They show that low-carb diets are more effective than traditional low-fat diets in lowering HbA1c, improving insulin sensitivity, reducing triglycerides, and promoting weight loss.

🥗 The most effective diet for diabetes is one that is "low in carbohydrates, rich in natural fats, and includes moderate protein—built around real, whole foods."

🍽 "Ideal Order of Eating for Blood Sugar Control":

1. "Fibre First" – Slows glucose absorption and reduces post-meal spikes. Best options include: simple green salads (cucumber, lettuce, methi), okra, cooked leafy greens, bottle gourd, flaxseed, chia seeds.
2. "Protein and Healthy Fats" – Help maintain satiety and blunt the glucose response.
3. "Unrefined Carbohydrates Last" – Always in small portions; best options include: red rice, rajmudi rice, millets, or steel-cut oats.

References

1. Means, C. (2024). Good Energy: The Surprising Link Between Metabolism and Health.
2. American Diabetes Association. (2024). Standards of Medical Care in Diabetes.
3. Feinman RD et al. (2015). Dietary carbohydrate restriction as the first approach in diabetes management. Nutrition, 31(1):1–13.
4. Westman EC et al. (2020). Low-carbohydrate nutrition and metabolism. The BMJ.
5. Unwin D, Unwin J. (2019). Low carbohydrate diet to achieve weight loss and improve HbA1c in type 2 diabetes. Diabetes Therapy.

CHAPTER 2

LOW CARB SCIENCE. HOW CUTTING CARBS CAN SEND DIABETES INTO REMISSION

What Is Diabetes Remission?

Diabetes remission is not a miracle—it's a medically defined, achievable state where HbA1c remains below 6.5% without glucose-lowering medications for at least 3–6 months.

How a Low-Carb Diet Works: The Metabolic Science

To understand how food induces remission, we must understand the metabolic traffic inside your body. A low-carb diet addresses glucose overload, insulin resistance, visceral fat, inflammation, and lipid dysfunction.

1. Reduces the Glucose Load

Carbohydrates, especially refined ones, are broken down into glucose—raising blood sugar levels. A low-carb diet minimizes glucose input and reduces post-meal hyperglycemia.

2. Lowers Insulin Demand

Low-carb diets reduce insulin secretion, restore insulin receptor sensitivity, and allow pancreatic beta cells to rest and recover.

3. Mobilizes Visceral Fat Stores

Low-carb eating reduces hepatic de novo lipogenesis, enhances lipolysis, and reverses liver and pancreatic fat—key factors in restoring metabolic health.

4. Reduces Inflammation and Oxidative Stress

Low-carb diets lower CRP, IL-6, TNF-alpha, and improve mitochondrial and endothelial function—reducing long-term damage.

5. Normalizes Lipid Profile and Triglycerides

Triglycerides drop significantly on low-carb diets; HDL rises; LDL particles shift to larger, less inflammatory forms.

Real-World Validation

Virta Health and the DiRECT trial provide international data. In India, over 100 patients in my practice have achieved remission using a structured low-carb approach.

Who Should Consider a Low-Carb Diet for Remission?

Ideal candidates include recent-onset diabetics, those with visceral fat or fatty liver, high fasting insulin, or multiple metabolic issues.

What a Remission Meal Plan Looks Like (Simplified)

Focus on real food: natural fats, adequate protein, non-starchy vegetables, and minimal unrefined carbs only when needed.

Important Reminders

Do not stop medications abruptly. Avoid extreme diets unsupervised. Monitor HbA1c, insulin, C-peptide, and lipids regularly. Customize for comorbidities.

Remission ≠ Cure

Diabetes remission is a fragile achievement that needs consistent dietary habits, monitoring, and support.

Real Case Study: A Turnaround at 50

Priya, a 42-year-old homemaker, achieved remission in 4 months with structured low-carb eating. Her medications were tapered, and remission has sustained over a year.

References

1. Hallberg SJ et al. (2018). Diabetes Therapy.
2. Athinarayanan SJ et al. (2019). Front Endocrinol.
3. Lean MEJ et al. (2018). The Lancet.
4. Ludwig DS, Ebbeling CB. (2021). Am J Clin Nutr.
5. Virta Health (2021). One-Year Outcomes Report.
6. ADA/EASD Consensus Report on Diabetes Remission (2022).

CHAPTER 3

THE POWER OF PROTEIN – THE MISSING LINK IN DIABETES MANAGEMENT

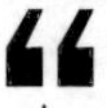

"Muscle is your metabolic engine. And protein is its fuel."

– Dr. Vishwanath BL

Protein is the most neglected macronutrient in diabetes care — yet it plays a central role in stabilizing blood sugar, supporting lean muscle mass, and improving satiety. However, its importance goes far beyond diabetes. A chronic protein-deficient diet can quietly disrupt metabolic health, immune resilience, and hormonal balance.

Protein Deficiency: A Hidden Driver of Metabolic Dysfunction

When protein intake is chronically low, the body breaks down muscle to compensate. This not only reduces resting metabolic rate but also worsens insulin resistance, creating a vicious cycle of weight gain, poor sugar control, and fatigue.

Protein deficiency is linked to:
– Loss of muscle mass (sarcopenia)
– Impaired immunity and frequent infections
– Poor wound healing
– Low energy and metabolic slowdown
– Sugar cravings and overeating
– Higher risk of fatty liver and visceral adiposity

The Protein Gap in Indian Diets

Surveys suggest more than 70% of Indians consume less than the recommended daily protein. Vegetarians and the elderly are particularly at risk. The most common Indian meals — rice, roti, dal — are high in carbohydrates and low in complete protein.

Symptoms of protein deficiency include fatigue, hair loss, poor muscle tone, sugar cravings, and frequent infections. Protein is critical not just for managing blood sugar but for overall cellular repair, hormone synthesis, and immune resilience.

Most Indian Breakfasts Are Protein-Poor

Popular Indian breakfasts like idli, dosa, upma, poha, or paratha are high in refined carbohydrates and low in protein. These meals often spike blood sugar and provide minimal satiety.

Instead, start the day with:
– Eggs or paneer bhurji
– Greek yogurt with seeds

– Moong chilla with chutney
– Protein smoothie with nuts and curd

Animal vs. Plant Protein: What Indians Need to Know

Animal proteins (eggs, fish, chicken, paneer) are complete proteins with all essential amino acids. Plant-based proteins (dal, legumes, nuts) are often incomplete unless combined properly. Vegetarians should prioritize:

– Whey protein
– Paneer
– Natural Greek yogurt
– Moong sprouts and soy
– Mixed pulses and seeds

Whey Protein: Myths and Facts

Myth: Whey is only for bodybuilders.

Fact: It is a complete, fast-absorbing protein ideal for vegetarians.

Myth: Whey damages kidneys.

Fact: Moderate use of whey protein is safe for healthy individuals.

Tip: Choose clean, reputable brands and avoid excessive intake. Whey should supplement — not replace — real food.

Don't Dump It All in One Meal

Many Indians eat most of their protein in one meal (e.g., Sunday biryani). The body can utilize only a limited protein at a time for muscle synthesis.

☑ Optimal strategy: Distribute protein across 3 meals, aiming for ~25–30g per meal. Goal: ~1g protein/kg body weight per day.

Why Healthcare Professionals Often Miss This

Many doctors and dietitians underemphasize protein due to limited nutrition training and outdated dietary guidelines. A study in the *Indian Journal of Medical Ethics* (2019) found fewer than 25% of Indian physicians had formal training in therapeutic nutrition.

Patients are often told to reduce fat and sugar, but rarely guided to improve protein intake. This misinformation delays metabolic improvement and diabetes remission.

Quick Recap

- Protein is crucial for blood sugar regulation, muscle health, and satiety
- Most Indian diets are protein-deficient, especially at breakfast
- Whey, paneer, and Greek yogurt are excellent options for vegetarians
- Spread protein throughout the day, not just one meal
- Misguided advice from healthcare professionals can hinder recovery

References

1. Indian Market Research Bureau (IMRB), 2020 – Protein Consumption in India
2. Layman DK (2004). Protein above the RDA improves body composition.

3. Joshi SR, JAPI (2019) – Nutrition and Diabetes.
4. Indian Journal of Medical Ethics, 2019 – Nutrition training in Indian medical curriculum.
5. Sathe A et al. (2021) – Protein gaps in Indian diets.

CHAPTER 4

THE LOW-FAT LIE – RETHINKING FATS IN DIABETES AND METABOLIC HEALTH

> "The fear of fat did more harm than fat itself."
>
> **– Dr. Vishwanath BL**

For years, health authorities promoted a low-fat diet as the gold standard for preventing heart disease and managing diabetes. This led to a public obsession with 'fat-free' products, many of which were high in sugar and refined carbohydrates. But modern science is now clear — not only is fat not the enemy, it is often essential for metabolic health and diabetes control.

Where Did the Low-Fat Idea Come From?

The idea that fat causes heart disease came from the flawed 'diet-heart hypothesis' in the 1960s. Despite limited evidence, it led to widespread promotion of low-fat, high-carb diets. This advice contributed to the rise of obesity and type 2 diabetes worldwide.

What Science Really Says About Dietary Fat

- The PURE study (2017) involving 135,000 people from 18 countries found that higher fat intake was associated with lower mortality, whereas high carbohydrate intake increased mortality risk.
- A 2020 meta-analysis in the Journal of the American College of Cardiology concluded that saturated fat is not significantly associated with heart disease.
- The Lancet (2017) review also showed that higher fat consumption — including saturated fat — was not linked to cardiovascular mortality.

Fat, Blood Sugar, and Metabolism

Dietary fat has minimal impact on blood sugar and insulin secretion. When consumed with carbs, fat slows down digestion, resulting in a lower glycemic response. This helps prevent post-meal sugar spikes.

Healthy fats support hormone production, brain function, cell membranes, and anti-inflammatory pathways. They also improve satiety, helping reduce overeating and aiding weight loss.

Healthy Fats to Include in Your Diet

- Ghee (clarified butter)
- Coconut and coconut oil
- Extra virgin olive oil

- Avocados
- Eggs (including yolks)
- Nuts and seeds: almonds, walnuts, chia, flaxseeds
- Paneer and full-fat curd

Unhealthy Fats to Avoid

- Refined vegetable oils (sunflower, soybean, corn oil)
- Hydrogenated fats and trans fats (found in packaged snacks, margarine)
- Repeatedly heated cooking oils (common in street food)

Busting Fat Myths

Myth: Fat causes weight gain

Fact: Excess sugar and refined carbs are more likely to cause fat storage.

Myth: Eating fat raises cholesterol and causes heart attacks

Fact: Healthy dietary fats — such as those from ghee, nuts, eggs, and olive oil — do not significantly raise blood cholesterol. Several large studies, including the PURE study and a 2020 JACC meta-analysis, have shown no strong correlation between natural fat intake and elevated LDL cholesterol. In fact, such fats may improve HDL (good cholesterol) and triglyceride profiles.

Quick Recap

- Low-fat diets are outdated and can worsen diabetes
- Healthy fats do not increase blood sugar
- Fats improve satiety and metabolic function

– Focus on natural fats; avoid refined vegetable oils and trans fats

References

1. Dehghan M, et al. (2017). Associations of fats and carbohydrate intake with cardiovascular disease and mortality in 18 countries. The Lancet.
2. Siri-Tarino PW, et al. (2020). Saturated fats and health: A reassessment and proposal for food-based recommendations. JACC.
3. Mozaffarian D, et al. (2006). Trans fatty acids and cardiovascular disease. NEJM.

CHAPTER 5

THE SUGAR THAT WASN'T SWEET — HOW HIDDEN CARBS SPIKE YOUR BLOOD SUGAR

When we think of sugar, we imagine sweets, desserts, colas, or white crystals on our table. But what if the most dangerous sugar isn't sweet at all?

Across India and the world, millions of people with diabetes avoid sweets religiously — yet their sugar readings remain high. The culprit often lies in everyday foods like rice, rotis, oats, fruits, or even "healthy" snacks. The truth is: your body doesn't care if sugar comes from a sweet or a starch. It only sees glucose.

The Myth of the "Non-Sweet" Meal

"I don't take sugar at all."

"I just had rice and dal."

"I had oats for dinner."

These are common phrases we hear from people struggling with their blood sugar. The problem? These foods are loaded with starch, which is just chains of glucose. The moment they're digested, they act just like sugar.

1 cup of cooked white rice can spike sugar just as much as 3 teaspoons of table sugar.

Understanding Glycemic Load (Not Just Glycemic Index)

The Glycemic Index (GI) tells us how quickly a food raises blood sugar. But it doesn't tell us how much sugar you actually get from a full portion. That's where Glycemic Load (GL) matters.

GL = GI x Carbohydrate amount in a portion / 100

Let's take an example:

- Watermelon has a high GI (~72), but low GL (because it has few carbs per serving)
- White rice has both high GI and high GL → double trouble

So even a "healthy" food can be risky if eaten in large quantities, or in isolation.

Top Indian Foods That Spike Sugar Quietly

Food Item	Problem
White rice	High GI + low fiber → quick spike

Chapati (atta)	Refined wheat, moderate GL, usually eaten in large quantities
Oats/Poha	High carb load, especially instant variants
Fruits in excess	Mangoes, bananas, grapes → high fructose and glucose
Fruit juices	Zero fiber, full sugar load hits the blood fast
Millets (when ground/fried)	Some raise sugar quickly if overprocessed
Protein bars/granola	Often sugar-rich, disguised with "natural" labels

Why Your Sugar Spikes Even Without Eating Sugar

- Too many carbs at one meal
- Lack of protein/fat in the meal
- Wrong meal sequencing (starting with rice/roti)
- Late-night eating → reduced insulin sensitivity
- Misleading labels (e.g., "no added sugar" but full of fruit puree, jaggery, honey)

What Helps Flatten the Curve?

1. Start your meal with fiber (salad/vegetables)
2. Include protein — paneer, eggs, tofu, whey shake
3. Add healthy fats — ghee, nuts, olive oil

4. Walk after meals — 10-15 minutes helps muscles soak up glucose
5. Control portion size — especially for rice, rotis, and cereals
6. Use lemon/vinegar — lowers meal glycemic response

The Real Danger: Chronic Spiking, Not Just One High Reading

It's not just about what your glucometer says 1 hour after eating. Frequent sugar spikes, even if temporary, increase:

- Oxidative stress
- Inflammation
- Risk of heart disease, nerve damage, kidney decline

That's why we must stop seeing carbs as "safe" just because they're not sweet.

Case 1: The Roti Trap

Mr. Ramesh, a 52-year-old accountant, had cut out sugar, desserts, and sweets for 6 months. Yet his post-meal sugar kept spiking above 220 mg/dL.

His typical lunch:

- 2 rotis
- Rice
- Dal
- Bhindi sabzi
- Buttermilk

What went wrong?

Though "no sweets" were consumed, his plate had over 60 grams of carbs in one meal — all rapidly digestible. There was no protein, no fat, and no fiber-first start.

Once he reduced one roti, added paneer, and began his meals with raw salad + a spoonful of ghee—his post-lunch sugar dropped to 160 mg/dL.

Case 2: The Smoothie Surprise

Neha, a 37-year-old IT professional, started her mornings with what she believed was a "super healthy" breakfast:

- A large smoothie made of banana, mango, dates, oats, almond milk, and a little honey.

Yet her sugar went from 95 (fasting) to 210 (1-hour post breakfast) despite no actual "sugar" added.

Why?

This "clean" smoothie was a bomb of hidden fructose and starch, with zero protein and no fiber buffering. Switching to a whey protein shake + almonds brought her post-meal spike down to 120.

Backed by Science

- A 2020 study in Diabetes Care showed that high post-meal glucose variability is a stronger predictor of complications than average glucose or fasting sugar.
- Japanese researchers found that eating vegetables and protein before rice reduced sugar spikes by 28–37%.

Quick Recap

- Sugar is not always sweet—it hides in starchy staples.
- The way you combine foods determines your sugar response.
- Meal sequencing, portion control, and protein save the day.
- Even "healthy" foods like oats and fruits can be problematic without balance.
- Real change comes from understanding how the body sees food, not how we taste it.

References

1. La Trobe University. Low-carb diet supported by a mobile app improved HbA1c and weight in T2DM patients. Herald Sun. 2025.
2. Jenkins DJA et al. Low Glycemic Index and Load Diets in T2DM: A review. 2024. PMC11519289.
3. Frontiers in Nutrition. Meal sequencing improves glycemic control in gestational diabetes. Front Nutr. 2024. 10.3389/fnut.2024.151.2231.
4. Translational Medicine. Glycemic variability and its association with complications in diabetes. BMC Transl Med. 2023.
5. Dong JY et al. Association between dietary glycemic index/load and risk of type 2 diabetes: A meta-analysis. 2023. PMC4144100.

CHAPTER 6

FACTS VS. FADS – DO TRADITIONAL REMEDIES LIKE ACV AND METHI REALLY WORK?

> "Science doesn't dismiss tradition. It tests it."
>
> – **Dr. Vishwanath BL**

1. The Indian Belief System Around Natural Remedies

Many Indians trust in the healing potential of traditional remedies like methi seeds, apple cider vinegar (ACV), jamun juice, amla, and karela. These beliefs are often passed down through generations and widely circulated through social media. But what does modern science say about their actual efficacy in controlling blood sugar?

2. Apple Cider Vinegar (ACV): What Science Says

Apple cider vinegar contains acetic acid, which slows gastric emptying and may improve insulin sensitivity. Studies have shown that consuming 1–2 tablespoons of ACV diluted in water before meals can significantly reduce post-meal glucose spikes.

✅ Benefits:

- Reduces post-meal sugar spikes by 20–30%
- Improves insulin sensitivity in short-term studies

❗ Caution:

- May irritate the throat or stomach if taken undiluted
- Not a replacement for medical treatment or lifestyle changes

3. Methi (Fenugreek) Seeds: Ancient Herb, Modern Evidence

Fenugreek seeds contain soluble fiber (galactomannan) and a compound called 4-hydroxyisoleucine that enhances insulin secretion. Traditionally soaked overnight and consumed on an empty stomach, methi has been shown to reduce fasting glucose and HbA1c in some studies.

✅ Benefits:

- Improves blood glucose control
- Enhances satiety and appetite regulation

4. Other Popular Indian Beliefs

Other traditional remedies include:

- "Jamun": Mild support for insulin sensitivity
- "Amla": Antioxidant-rich, helps in reducing oxidative stress
- "Cinnamon": May help lower fasting glucose (Ceylon type preferred)

– "Karela Juice": Anecdotal support, weak evidence, and poor palatability

5. Should You Use These Remedies?

These remedies may serve as helpful adjuncts to a structured lifestyle and medication plan. However, they should not be considered standalone treatments. Discussing them with your healthcare provider is essential to ensure they fit safely into your diabetes management strategy.

6. Quick Recap

– ACV and methi seeds have moderate scientific backing for controlling sugar spikes
– Use traditional remedies as supportive measures, not cures
– Always consult a healthcare provider before integrating them into your regimen
– Traditional wisdom and science can work hand in hand, when used wisely

References

1. Johnston CS et al. (2004). Vinegar improves insulin sensitivity to a high-carbohydrate meal. Diabetes Care.
2. Neelakantan N et al. (2014). Effect of fenugreek on glycemia: A meta-analysis. Nutrition Journal.
3. Akilen R et al. (2010). Cinnamon in type 2 diabetes: A systematic review. Annals of Family Medicine.
4. Indian Council of Medical Research Guidelines on Complementary Therapies in Diabetes, 2022.

CHAPTER 7

SEED OILS AND SUGAR SPIKES – THE HIDDEN LINK IN YOUR KITCHEN

> "What you fry your food in could be spiking your sugars more than what you fry."

The Oil We Forgot to Question

Sugar is always the villain. Rice is blamed. Even fruits get scrutinized. But what about the oil in our food — the one we use every single day?

Walk into most Indian homes, and you'll find bottles of sunflower, safflower, rice bran, soybean, or canola oil — proudly labeled "heart-healthy." We were told these were modern, light, and cholesterol-free. But behind the clarity of these refined oils lies a murky truth — one that affects your inflammation, insulin resistance, and sugar control.

Yes, your diabetes may be silently simmering in your frying pan.

What Are Seed Oils, Really?

Seed oils are extracted from the seeds of crops — not from fruits or nuts — using high heat, chemical solvents (like hexane), and then refined, bleached, and deodorized. The result is a clear, odorless oil with a long shelf life. But there's a trade-off — and it's steep.

These oils are:

- Rich in omega-6 polyunsaturated fats (especially linoleic acid)
- Easily oxidized when heated
- Low in natural antioxidants
- Often used repeatedly in Indian cooking (think: frying pooris, bhajjis, pakoras)

Why Are They a Problem for Diabetics?

1. They Fuel Chronic Inflammation

Excess omega-6 fats from seed oils tilt the body toward inflammation — a low-grade, persistent fire within your cells that:

- Increases insulin resistance
- Slows down sugar metabolism
- Encourages fatty liver
- Makes you feel bloated, tired, and foggy

2. They're Highly Unstable When Heated

Indian cooking often involves high temperatures—tadkas, deep frying, and roasting. When seed oils are heated repeatedly (or even once), they produce toxic byproducts like:

- Aldehydes (e.g., acrolein, 4-HNE)
- Free radicals
- Trans fats (in trace amounts)

These damage your pancreatic beta cells, impair mitochondrial function, and worsen glucose tolerance, quietly chipping away at your ability to reverse or control diabetes.

3. They Disrupt Gut and Metabolic Health

Emerging science suggests that high intake of linoleic acid may:

- Alter the gut microbiome
- Increase gut permeability ("leaky gut")
- Allow toxins (like LPS) to enter the bloodstream

This leads to metabolic endotoxemia — a fancy term for toxins triggering inflammation and insulin resistance from the inside out.

The Indian Trap

We stopped using traditional fats like ghee, cold-pressed coconut oil, or mustard oil, thinking they were "heavy" or "unhealthy." But we replaced them with industrial oils that were never part of our cultural diet.

What we didn't realize:

- The average Indian now consumes 10x more omega-6 than omega-3
- Street food, packaged snacks, biscuits, and namkeens are all loaded with reused seed oils

– Even health-conscious households often use "refined oil blends" that do more harm than good

So, What Oils Should Diabetics Use?

You don't need fancy imported oils. You need traditional wisdom, restored. Here's a simple guide:

Oil	Best Use	Why It Works
Desi Ghee	Cooking, tadka, low-heat frying	Butyrate-rich, anti-inflammatory, stabilizes blood sugar
Cold-Pressed Coconut Oil	High-heat cooking	Saturated fat, resistant to oxidation
Cold-Pressed Mustard Oil	Everyday Indian cooking	Rich in MUFA, low omega-6, natural antioxidants
Groundnut Oil (Unrefined)	Medium-heat cooking	Balanced fat profile
Virgin Olive Oil	Salads, light sautéing	High in heart-healthy MUFAs

Kitchen Swaps That Heal

– Replace refined sunflower/rice bran oil with cold-pressed coconut oil or mustard oil
– Use ghee generously in dals, rotis, and vegetables

- Stop reusing oil from fried snacks
- Switch from store-bought snacks to roasted nuts or seeds
- Limit restaurant fried food — it's a PUFA trap

Final Message

For decades, fat was wrongly blamed for heart disease and diabetes. But the real enemy is poor-quality, industrial fat—not traditional fat.

In a diabetic kitchen, what matters is not just how much fat you eat, but what kind.

Sugar may spike you fast.

Seed oils damage you slowly.

And sometimes, it's the slow burn that does the most harm.

📚 Suggested References

1. DiNicolantonio JJ, O'Keefe JH. The dark side of vegetable oils. Open Heart. 2018;5(2):e000898.
2. Ramsden CE, Zamora D, Leelarthaepin B, et al. Use of dietary linoleic acid for secondary prevention of coronary heart disease. BMJ. 2013;346:e8707.
3. Fritsche KL. The science of fatty acids and inflammation. Adv Nutr. 2015;6(3):293S–301S.
4. Ghosh S, Chatterjee S. Studies on oxidative stability and shelf-life of selected edible oils in India. J Food Sci Technol. 2021;58(5):1803–1810.

5. Kothari D, Patel S, Kim SK. Prospective uses of plant-derived oils in clinical and therapeutic practices: a review. Biomed Pharmacother. 2022;149:112890.
6. Narang R, Gupta N, Bhatla M, et al. Comparative evaluation of mustard oil and sunflower oil on glycemic and lipid parameters in patients with type 2 diabetes mellitus. Indian J Endocrinol Metab. 2021;25(1):40–46.

CHAPTER 8

CAN YOU EAT LESS AND HEAL MORE?

Intermittent Fasting and the Return to India's Forgotten Rhythms

For centuries, Indians practiced fasting not as a weight loss trend, but as a discipline of health, clarity, and devotion. Whether it was Ekadashi, Ramzan, Navratri, or even simple evening temple customs, food was never constant. Eating windows were limited. Mindful. Purposeful.

Today, science calls it intermittent fasting, and what was once tradition is now being rediscovered as one of the most powerful tools to reverse insulin resistance, inflammation, and metabolic disease.

What Is Intermittent Fasting, Really?

It's not starvation. It's structured eating with planned periods of no food. The most common types include:

- Time-Restricted Eating (TRE): Eat in an 8–10 hour window (e.g., 10 am to 6 pm)

- 16:8 Fasting: 16 hours fast, 8 hours eating
- 5:2 Method: 2 low-calorie days per week
- 24-Hour Fast: Once a week or fortnight

Fasting works not by reducing calories alone, but by shifting hormonal gears.

The Metabolic Benefits

- Reduces insulin levels → gives cells a break from constant sugar overload
- Boosts fat burning → once glucose depletes, body taps into fat
- Improves insulin sensitivity → key in reversing type 2 diabetes
- Triggers autophagy → body cleans up damaged cells
- Reduces inflammation and triglycerides
- Improves sleep, cognition, gut repair

A 2023 Indian study showed that 14:10 and 16:8 fasting improved HbA1c, weight, and liver enzymes within 3 months, without additional medications.

Traditional Indian Rhythms Were Already Fasting-Optimized

- No meals before sunrise or after sunset in many customs
- Upvas (fasting) once a week — on Mondays, Thursdays, Ekadashi
- Skipping grains or sugars on certain days
- Temple offerings before the first bite → natural delay in eating
- Seasonal fasts → detox, digestion reset

Our ancestors were unintentionally following time-restricted eating, aligned with circadian biology.

Common Myths That Are Holding Indians Back

Myth	Truth
You must eat every 2–3 hours	This spikes insulin repeatedly and leads to fatigue. Your body thrives in rest-digest cycles.
Breakfast is the most important meal	For diabetics, skipping early meals may reduce glucose load.
Fasting causes ulcers	Fasting with hydration does not cause ulcers. Stress and H. pylori do.
You'll faint without carbs	The body has fuel reserves (glycogen, fat). Transition can feel weak at first, but adapts fast.

Case Study: From Glucose Rollercoaster to Gentle Curve

Mrs. Lakshmi, 48, had fasting sugars of 140–150 despite walking and no sweets.

She shifted to a 16:8 eating window (10:30 am–6:30 pm). First meals: dal + salad + paneer.

No food post 7 pm. Early dinners with family.

Result in 2 months:

- Fasting sugar dropped to 102
- 3 kg weight loss
- No change in medications
- Reported better sleep, focus, and digestion

How to Start (Without Feeling Deprived)

1. Delay breakfast by 1 hour every 3–4 days
2. Finish dinner earlier — target 6:30–7:00 pm
3. Stay hydrated — lemon water, herbal teas, black coffee (no sugar)
4. Ensure enough protein and fat to avoid hunger pangs
5. Avoid breaking fast with sugar or rice—start with protein
6. Begin with 12:12 or 14:10 before jumping to 16:8
7. Skip a meal when not hungry—that's wisdom, not weakness

Quick Recap

- Intermittent fasting isn't new—it's India's old wisdom, repackaged
- Fasting reduces insulin, improves metabolism, and reverses sugar imbalance
- Start small: shorten your eating window gradually
- Focus on what breaks your fast: protein > carbs
- Fasting isn't starvation—it's metabolic rest and repair

CHAPTER 9

FASTING SAFELY — WHAT EVERY DIABETIC MUST KNOW BEFORE SKIPPING A MEAL

Fasting, when done right, can be a powerful tool for blood sugar control and metabolic healing. But for people with diabetes—especially those on medications—fasting without preparation can lead to dangerous consequences like hypoglycemia, fatigue, and hospitalization.

This chapter provides a science-backed, easy-to-follow guide on how diabetics can fast safely. It also highlights when fasting might not be advisable.

Why Fasting Needs Caution in Diabetes

Fasting alters your usual glucose metabolism. In diabetics taking medications like insulin or sulfonylureas, skipping meals can lead to sharp drops in blood sugar.

The risk includes:

- Hypoglycemia (blood sugar <70 mg/dL)
- Dizziness, sweating, confusion, fainting
- Rebound hyperglycemia due to overcorrection
- Diabetic ketoacidosis in Type 1 DM (rare but serious)

This is why fasting must be individualized based on your medications, glucose patterns, and overall health.

Who Should NOT Fast

- Type 1 diabetes with poor sugar control
- Pregnant or breastfeeding women
- Elderly diabetics with comorbidities
- Diabetics with a history of recurrent hypoglycemia
- Advanced kidney or liver disease
- Unstable cardiac patients

Always consult your physician before beginning any fasting regimen.

Medication-Specific Guidance

1. "Metformin": Safe during fasting. Usually, no dose change is needed.
2. "Sulfonylureas (e.g., glimepiride, gliclazide)": High risk of hypoglycemia. May require dose reduction or avoidance during fasting.
3. "Insulin": Basal insulin may be continued with dose adjustments. Bolus insulin should be skipped or reduced during meal-skipping.

4. "DPP-4 inhibitors (e.g., sitagliptin)": Generally safe. Minimal risk of hypoglycemia.
5. "SGLT2 inhibitors": Watch for dehydration. Ensure adequate fluid intake. May be withheld on prolonged fasts.
6. "GLP-1 receptor agonists": Often compatible but can suppress appetite. Monitor sugar.

"Note": Adjustments must always be supervised by a healthcare professional.

Monitoring During Fasting

- Use CGM (Continuous Glucose Monitoring) or check sugars at home using a glucometer.
- Suggested check times: before breaking fast, 2 hours after meals, at bedtime.
- Break your fast immediately if blood sugar < 70 mg/dL or you feel symptomatic.
- Stay well hydrated, especially in warm climates or longer fasts.
- Include electrolyte-rich fluids like buttermilk, lime water, or salt water if prolonged.

Smart Fasting for Diabetics

- Prefer time-restricted eating (TRE): Start with 12:12 and progress to 14:10
- Always eat a protein-rich meal before a prolonged fast
- Avoid sugary foods when breaking the fast — go for proteins and fiber first
- Add a little ghee or healthy fat to stabilize sugars

- Avoid fasting for more than 16 hours without medical supervision

Case Example: Safe Ramadan Fasting with Insulin

Mr. Ahmed, a 58-year-old man with type 2 diabetes on insulin glargine and glimepiride, wanted to fast during Ramadan.

With doctor guidance:

- His insulin dose was reduced by 20%
- Glimepiride was stopped temporarily
- He monitored sugars 4 times a day
- Meals were shifted to suhoor (pre-dawn) and iftar (post-sunset)

He completed 27 fasts safely. No hypoglycemia episodes. Lost 3 kg and reduced HbA1c by 0.6% in 6 weeks.

Quick Recap

- Diabetics can fast safely, but not without planning.
- Medication dose, type, and timing must be adjusted.
- Monitor sugar levels regularly and know when to break the fast.
- Certain groups (pregnant, elderly, Type 1, CKD) should avoid fasting.
- Consult your physician before making any changes.

References

1. International Diabetes Federation. (2023). Diabetes and Ramadan: Practical Guidelines.

2. American Diabetes Association (ADA). Standards of Medical Care in Diabetes—2024.
3. Joshi SR et al. (2022). Safe Fasting Practices in Type 2 Diabetes Mellitus. JAPI.
4. Malinowski B et al. (2023). Intermittent fasting in diabetes mellitus type 2. Nutrients.
5. Kalra S et al. (2023). Guidelines for insulin use during religious fasting in South Asians. Int J Clin Pract.

CHAPTER 10

SMART SUPPLEMENTING – WHAT EVERY DIABETIC SHOULD (AND SHOULDN'T) TAKE

Supplements are not shortcuts to good health, but when used wisely, they can be powerful tools in the diabetic toolkit. Due to dietary gaps, medication side effects, and modern food processing, many people with diabetes are deficient in key nutrients. This chapter guides you through essential supplements that support blood sugar control, metabolic health, and overall well-being.

"You can't supplement your way out of a bad diet. But you can fill the cracks with the right choices."

💊 Why Supplements Matter in Diabetes

People with diabetes, especially in India, often have undiagnosed deficiencies in Vitamin D, B12, magnesium, and omega-3 fatty acids. These deficits affect energy, nerve function, insulin sensitivity, and cardiovascular health. Medications like metformin further deplete key vitamins like B12. Supplements, taken under proper medical advice, help correct these gaps.

📋 Key Supplements for Diabetics

- Vitamin D: Improves insulin sensitivity and reduces inflammation Recommended Form: Cholecalciferol (D3) How to Take: Take weekly (60,000 IU) or daily (2000 IU) based on levels

- Vitamin B12: Protects nerves, especially in those on metformin Recommended Form: Methylcobalamin How to Take: Sublingual or IM injections if deficient
- Magnesium: Enhances insulin function, sleep, and muscle recovery Recommended Form: Magnesium Glycinate or Citrate How to Take: Avoid oxide form; take at night
- Alpha-Lipoic Acid (ALA): Antioxidant; relieves diabetic neuropathy Recommended Form: R-ALA How to Take: Take on an empty stomach
- Omega-3 Fatty Acids: Supports heart health and lowers triglycerides Recommended Form: EPA + DHA from fish oil or krill oil How to Take: Choose enteric-coated forms
- Zinc: Improves glucose metabolism and immune support Recommended Form: Zinc Picolinate or Citrate How to Take: 15–30 mg/day
- Probiotics: Improves gut health, metabolism, and inflammation Recommended Form: Lactobacillus, Bifidobacterium strains How to Take: Look for 10–50 billion CFUs

- Multivitamins: Covers general micronutrient deficiencies Recommended Form: Diabetic-specific formulations How to Take: Choose one with B-complex, D, C, zinc, selenium

⚠ How to Take Supplements Safely

- Always consult a physician or dietician before starting any supplement.
- Do not overdose on fat-soluble vitamins (A, D, E, K) — they can build up in the body.
- Track your blood levels (e.g., Vitamin D, B12, magnesium) before and during supplementation.
- Take probiotics on an empty stomach or as directed.
- Supplements are "not" replacements for a poor diet — they work best alongside a balanced, nutrient-rich meal plan.

🚫 Popular But Questionable Supplements

- Chromium – Limited consistent benefit in clinical trials.
- Bitter melon extract – Better taken in natural form with meals.
- Ayurvedic mixes – Often lack standardization and can interact with medications.

🔁 Quick Recap

- Supplements help fill nutritional gaps in diabetes management, but should not replace a healthy diet.
- Key supplements include Vitamin D, B12, Magnesium, ALA, Omega-3, Zinc, Probiotics, and Diabetic Multivitamins.
- Choose the right form of each supplement and consult a doctor before starting.

- Avoid self-medicating with herbal mixes or unverified supplements claiming to 'cure' diabetes.
- Supplements work best when combined with good nutrition, lifestyle, and regular blood sugar monitoring.

References

1. American Diabetes Association. Standards of Medical Care in Diabetes—2025. Diabetes Care. 2025;48(Suppl 1):S1–S200.
2. Bailey CJ, et al. Metformin and vitamin B12 deficiency: assessment and management. Diabetes Obes Metab. 2023;25(1):234–240.
3. Veronese N, et al. Magnesium and health outcomes: A meta-analysis. Br J Nutr. 2024;131(4):489–498.
4. Diniz Vilela DF, et al. Effects of probiotics on glycemic control: A systematic review and meta-analysis. Clin Nutr. 2023;42(2):357–365.
5. Indian Council of Medical Research (ICMR). Micronutrient Gaps in Indian Adults. ICMR Report, 2023.

SECTION 4

LIFESTYLE AS A MEDICINE – DAILY ROUTINE THAT HEALS

CHAPTER 1

LIFESTYLE IS THE LIFELINE – DAILY HABITS THAT CHANGE EVERYTHING

Why Medication Alone Is Not Enough

Medications can help lower blood sugar levels, but they don't reverse the root cause of type 2 diabetes — insulin resistance. True healing comes when you stop feeding the disease and start supporting your body's natural metabolic balance. That happens through lifestyle, not just prescriptions.

Nutrition: Eat to Lower Sugar and Insulin

Nutrition is the most powerful tool in managing and even reversing insulin resistance. The goal is not just to control blood sugar, but to lower the body's overall insulin demand. When you eat to reduce both glucose spikes and chronic hyperinsulinemia, you give your body the best chance to heal.

Movement: Muscles Are Sugar Sponges

Physical activity is medicine. After meals, walking helps muscles absorb glucose directly. But the real game-changer is "resistance training".

Lifting weights "2–3 times a week" builds muscle, improves insulin sensitivity, and raises your resting metabolic rate. It's especially important for people over 40 who are losing muscle mass every year.

Small daily movements—stretching, walking meetings, climbing stairs—add up and keep glucose in check.

Sleep: Your Hormonal Reset Button

Poor sleep increases hunger, cortisol, and insulin resistance. Many diabetics also suffer from sleep apnea, which worsens blood sugar control.

Aim for "7–8 hours of restorative sleep" per night. Create a wind-down routine, reduce screen time before bed, and keep your sleep schedule consistent.

Stress: The Invisible Spike

Chronic stress leads to elevated cortisol, which raises blood sugar levels even without food. Stress also disrupts sleep, increases cravings, and worsens insulin resistance.

Use techniques like "yoga", "mindfulness", "breathing exercises", and "digital detoxes".

🙏 As Buddha taught: *"A calm mind leads to a healthy body."* He emphasized that mental agitation creates physical suffering, and that true healing begins within.

Fasting and Circadian Rhythm

Fasting gives your body time to reset, reduce insulin levels, and improve metabolic flexibility. Aligning your meals with natural hormonal rhythms—such as finishing dinner early and avoiding late-night snacks—can support better glucose control. Practices like "Time-Restricted Eating (TRE)", where meals are consumed within an 8–10 hour window, have been shown to lower insulin resistance and inflammation.

⚠ Fasting for individuals with diabetes, especially those on medications or insulin, should always be done under medical supervision.

🕊 Many religious traditions — including Hinduism, Islam, Buddhism, and Christianity — incorporate fasting as a means of physical and spiritual discipline. Modern science now supports these practices as beneficial for metabolic health when applied correctly and safely.

Fasting doesn't mean starvation—it means giving your body time to recover.

An "overnight fast of 12–14 hours" allows insulin levels to drop and the body to switch to fat-burning mode. Eating earlier in the evening aligns with natural hormonal rhythms.

"Time-restricted eating (TRE)" improves insulin sensitivity, lowers inflammation, and promotes better metabolic control.

Doctor's Take

The most dramatic results I've seen came not from new medications, but from daily routine changes. Patients who prioritize food, movement, sleep, and emotional balance often reduce or stop medications entirely. Lifestyle doesn't just support healing—it drives it.

Quick Recap

- Medications help manage blood sugar but do not reverse insulin resistance.
- Low-carb, high-fiber, protein-rich diets reduce insulin load and hunger.
- Weight training 2–3x/week significantly improves insulin sensitivity.
- Sleep and stress management are essential for metabolic healing.
- Fasting and aligning meals with circadian rhythm enhances hormonal balance.

References

1. American Diabetes Association. Standards of Medical Care in Diabetes—2024. Diabetes Care.
2. Roy Taylor. The Twin Cycle Hypothesis for Type 2 Diabetes. Diabetologia, 2018.

3. Means, Casey. Good Energy: The Surprising Connection Between Metabolism and Health. 2024.
4. Indian Council of Medical Research (ICMR). STW for Type 2 Diabetes Mellitus, 2022.
5. Longo, V., & Panda, S. Fasting, Circadian Rhythms, and Time-Restricted Feeding in Healthy Lifespan. Cell Metabolism, 2016.

CHAPTER 2

MOVE LIKE YOUR ANCESTORS – REDISCOVERING NATURAL EXERCISE

> “Movement is our ancestral medicine.
> Stillness is the modern disease.”
>
> **– Dr. Vishwanath BL**

Our bodies were never designed for long hours of sitting or screen time. For thousands of years, human life involved walking, squatting, climbing, carrying, and active labor. Modern diabetes isn't just about diet — it's about a lack of ancestral movement. Even brief periods of activity, like a 10-minute post-meal walk, can dramatically improve glucose control and insulin sensitivity.

Move Like Your Ancestors

Here's how traditional Indian lifestyles inspired movements that are still powerful today:

- 🏞 "Barefoot or outdoor walking": Walking on natural terrain like grass or soil strengthens foot muscles, enhances balance, and improves glucose metabolism. It also connects your body to the Earth—a process called grounding—which research suggests can reduce inflammation, lower stress hormones, and improve blood circulation.
- 🧘 "Squatting": Traditional cooking, praying, and eating involved deep squats. This posture improves hip mobility and leg strength.
- ⊠ "Lifting and carrying": From fetching water to farming, our ancestors built strength naturally. You can replicate this with dumbbells or resistance bands.
- 🌞 "Surya Namaskar & yoga": These time-honored practices improve flexibility, circulation, and insulin sensitivity.
- 🤼 "Playing traditional games": Activities like kho-kho or kabaddi involve sprinting and agility, perfect for blood sugar regulation.

Walking: Balance Brisk with Mindful

Modern science now confirms what ancient wisdom practiced: walking heals. The best approach? Combine both brisk and mindful walking in equal measure:

- "Brisk Walking (50%)": Speeds up your heart rate, helps burn calories, and significantly lowers post-meal glucose spikes.
- "Mindful Walking (50%)": Practiced in Buddhism, it involves slow, aware steps with full focus on breathing. Buddha recommended this not just for physical health, but to calm

the mind and reduce mental suffering—a key driver of high cortisol and poor glucose control.

Integrating both types of walking brings balance: metabolic fitness from brisk walking and hormonal harmony from mindfulness.

Strength Is the New Sugar Sponge

Muscle acts like a sponge for sugar. Traditional lifestyles involved physical labor that kept muscles strong and insulin sensitivity high. Today, resistance training just 2–3 times a week can mimic that effect.

- Do squats, push-ups, or resistance band exercises
- Start light and build consistently
- Focus on large muscle groups—legs, back, and core

Are 10,000 Steps Necessary?

The idea of 10,000 steps a day began as a marketing campaign but has since found scientific support. Studies show that even 6,000 to 8,000 steps daily can reduce the risk of heart disease, diabetes, and premature death.

If you're managing diabetes, aim for post-meal walks and general movement throughout the day. Don't stress the number—consistency is more important than perfection.

Quick Recap

- Move like your ancestors: walk, squat, carry, stretch, and play
- Balance your daily walks: 50% brisk, 50% mindful
- Practice Surya Namaskar or yoga for strength and stress control

- Add strength training twice or thrice a week
- Aim for 6,000–10,000 steps/day—not mandatory, but ideal
- The best exercise is the one you'll keep doing daily

References

1. Ekelund, U. et al. (2019). 'Dose-response associations between accelerometry measured physical activity and sedentary time and all cause mortality: systematic review and harmonised meta-analysis.' BMJ, 366:l4570.
2. Colberg, S. R. et al. (2016). 'Exercise and Type 2 Diabetes: The American College of Sports Medicine and the American Diabetes Association joint position statement.' Diabetes Care, 39(11):2065-2079.
3. Dempsey, P. C. et al. (2016). 'Interrupting prolonged sitting reduces postprandial glucose and insulin responses.' Diabetes Care, 39(6):964-972.
4. Hall, K. S. et al. (2020). 'Steps per Day and Mortality in Older Adults in the US.' JAMA, 323(12):1151-1160.

CHAPTER 3

SLEEP, STRESS & SUGAR — THE UNSEEN AXIS

In the lives of millions managing diabetes, it's easy to focus on food, exercise, and medications, but often miss what happens in the quiet hours of the night, or in the mental storms no one sees. Sleep and stress are not secondary—they are foundational to glucose control and long-term health.

Let's uncover how two invisible forces—rest and unrest—influence every drop of sugar in your bloodstream.

Sleep: The Natural Insulin Booster

Sleep isn't passive. It's when your brain detoxes, hormones reset, and metabolism aligns. But with late-night screens, urban noise, and anxiety, restorative sleep is now a luxury for many.

Research shows:

- Poor sleep reduces insulin sensitivity—your body struggles to use insulin, leading to higher sugars.
- Even partial sleep deprivation for just a week can elevate fasting glucose to prediabetic levels.

– Deep sleep helps regulate ghrelin and leptin, hormones that control hunger and satiety. When disrupted, we crave more and eat more—often at night.

A study published in *The Lancet* (1999) found that just 6 nights of 4-hour sleep in healthy adults led to significant glucose intolerance.

Stress: The Invisible Sugar Spike

Stress is not just emotional; it's hormonal. Whether it's deadlines, illness, caregiving, or loneliness—your body doesn't differentiate. It responds by releasing cortisol and adrenaline, both of which raise blood sugar.

Effects of chronic stress:
– Increases glucose production by the liver
– Promotes central fat gain (especially belly fat)
– Worsens insulin resistance
– Encourages late-night eating and sleep disruption

The same hormones that save your life in an emergency can slowly damage your metabolism when always "on."

Chronic stress activates the HPA axis, leading to elevated cortisol—a known diabetogenic hormone.

The Stress–Sleep–Sugar Loop

The relationship is cyclical:
– Stress reduces sleep quality.
– Poor sleep increases emotional reactivity.
– Both raise cortisol.

– Cortisol elevates blood glucose.

This creates a loop where mental health and metabolic health deteriorate together.

Breaking this loop isn't about perfection. It's about small, steady changes.

Quick Recap

- Even mild sleep loss can impair insulin sensitivity and raise blood sugar.
- Chronic stress stimulates hormonal pathways that worsen glucose control.
- These effects are often independent of diet or physical activity.
- Restoring sleep and reducing stress can significantly improve metabolic markers.
- A calm evening mind supports better glucose levels by morning.

References

1. Spiegel K et al. Impact of Sleep Debt on Metabolic and Endocrine Function. Lancet. 1999;354(9188):1435–1439.
2. Van Cauter E et al. Sleep and Metabolism: An Overview. Sleep Med Clin. 2007;2(2):147–162.
3. Black PH. The Stress Response and Inflammation. J R Soc Med. 1994;87(8):500–504.
4. Walker M. Why We Sleep. Penguin, 2017.

CHAPTER 4

THE YOGIC PRESCRIPTION – ANCIENT PRACTICE, MODERN DIABETES CURE

Yoga is far more than a form of exercise—it is a complete science of life. Originating in ancient India, yoga is a discipline of physical postures, controlled breathing, internal cleansing, and meditative stillness. When practiced mindfully and consistently under proper guidance, yoga has the potential to awaken the innate healer within you. For people with diabetes, yoga offers a holistic, side-effect-free approach to improving insulin sensitivity, balancing stress hormones, and rejuvenating the body's metabolic systems.

Modern research now recognizes what ancient yogic texts claimed centuries ago—diabetes can be significantly improved, and in some cases reversed, through yogic practices. This chapter outlines how yoga supports metabolic health and provides a curated set of postures and practices beneficial for those living with diabetes.

5 Ways Yoga Supports Diabetes Management and Reversal

1. Stimulates the Pancreas: Many yoga asanas (postures) involve abdominal compression and release, which enhances blood and oxygen flow to the pancreas.
2. Balances Endocrine Glands: Certain postures, pranayama (breathing practices), and meditation stabilize hormonal output from the thyroid, adrenal glands, and pancreas.
3. Improves Glucose Uptake by Muscles: Yoga increases muscular glucose absorption independent of insulin.
4. Reduces Chronic Stress: Cortisol, the stress hormone, plays a significant role in raising blood sugar. Yoga activates the parasympathetic nervous system.
5. Builds Mental Clarity and Discipline: Regular yoga enhances focus, self-awareness, and lifestyle adherence.

The Yogic Framework for Diabetes Management

A complete yogic approach includes:

- Sattvic Aahara – A clean, plant-based, whole-food diet rooted in yogic philosophy.
- Asanas – Specific postures that stimulate metabolism and internal organs.
- Kriyas – Cleansing techniques that detoxify and improve gut health.
- Pranayama – Breathing techniques to regulate energy and stress.
- Bandhas – Neuromuscular locks for hormonal balance.
- Meditation – Mindfulness practices to cultivate inner awareness and calm.

Best Yoga Asanas for Diabetes: The 6-Posture Module

- Padahastasana (Standing Forward Bend): Increases blood flow to the pancreas. Contraindicated in pregnancy.
- Ardha Matsyendrasana (Seated Spinal Twist): Stimulates the pancreas and digestive organs. Avoid during pregnancy.
- Paschimottanasana (Seated Forward Bend): Massages abdominal viscera, regulates digestion.
- Dhanurasana (Bow Pose): Strengthens back muscles and tones abdominal organs. Avoid during pregnancy and severe back pain.
- Mandukasana (Frog Pose): Activates the pancreas and improves insulin output. Not recommended during pregnancy.
- Sarvangasana (Shoulder Stand): Improves endocrine function. Avoid in pregnancy, hypertension, and diabetic heart complications.

3 High-Impact Yogic Practices for Diabetes

- Kapalabhati: A cleansing breath that contracts abdominal muscles, enhancing insulin sensitivity.
- Agnisara Kriya: Rapid flapping of abdominal muscles while breath is held out; tones the gut and stimulates insulin production.
- Surya Namaskar: Combines movement, breath, and gratitude. Enhances circulation, detox, and metabolic health.

Precautions and Guidance

– Learn under a trained yoga therapist, especially if on medications.

- Avoid inversion postures in heart disease, hypertension, or complications like retinopathy.
- Pregnant women should skip deep twists and intense pranayama.
- Consult your physician before starting yoga if you're on medications that may cause hypoglycemia.

Final Thoughts: A Mind-Body Phenomenon

Yoga is not merely a workout—it is a spiritual, biochemical, and emotional recalibration. When practiced with awareness, it awakens the body's innate healing intelligence. From a yogic perspective, diabetes is not just a sugar problem—it's a disruption of internal harmony. By aligning breath, body, and awareness, yoga brings balance to the metabolic orchestra, one asana at a time.

"When the abdominal energy center is activated and the inner channels are purified, the body becomes free of disease."

References

1. Innes KE, Vincent HK. The influence of yoga-based programs on risk profiles in adults with type 2 diabetes mellitus: A systematic review. Evid Based Complement Alternat Med. 2007.
2. Satish R, Raju TR. Efficacy of yoga in the control of type 2 diabetes mellitus. J Indian Med Assoc. 2002.
3. Jyotsna VP, Joshi A, Ambekar S, Kumar N, Sreenivas V. Comprehensive yogic breathing program improves quality

of life in patients with diabetes. Indian J Endocrinol Metab. 2012.

4. American Diabetes Association. Physical activity/exercise and diabetes: Position statement. Diabetes Care. 2016.
5. Bhavanani AB. Role of yoga in prevention and management of diabetes. J Yoga Phys Ther. 2013.

— Hatha Yoga Pradipika, Chapter 2, Verse 4

CHAPTER 5

STRONGER MUSCLES, STRONGER METABOLISM – RESISTANCE TRAINING FOR DIABETES CONTROL

The Indian Reality

In India, most individuals with type 2 diabetes—especially those over 45 or 50—consider walking their default mode of exercise...

What Is Resistance Training?

Resistance training (also known as strength training or weight training) involves using external resistance...

Scientific Benefits of Strength Training in Diabetes

- Improves Insulin Sensitivity – better than aerobic activity in some cases.
- Increases Glucose Utilization – even at rest, helping maintain stable blood sugar.

- Reduces Fat-to-Muscle Ratio – improves insulin sensitivity and reduces inflammation.
- Strengthens Bones & Prevents Falls – especially for postmenopausal women.
- Boosts Basal Metabolic Rate – facilitates easier weight control.
- Delays Aging – improves mitochondrial function and slows biological decline.
- Enhances Functional Independence – supports daily tasks and mobility.

Weekly Plan for Diabetics

A balanced plan should ideally include:
– 3 days/week of aerobic activity (e.g., brisk walking, cycling)
– 2 days/week of resistance training

Sample Beginner Strength Training Routine

- Planks – Core stabilization
- Squats – Lower body and glutes
- Lunges – Functional balance
- Standing Biceps Curls – Arm strength
- Triceps Extensions – Arm and shoulder tone
- Shoulder Presses – Upper body strength
- Chest Press – Push strength (machine or floor)
- Classic Crunches – Abdominal/core strength

Tips for Safe & Effective Training

- Always warm up and mobilize joints before lifting.
- Progress gradually with repetitions and resistance.

- Use a combination of resistance bands, machines, and free weights.
- Work with a certified fitness trainer if new to strength training.
- Monitor your body's response: fatigue, soreness, and energy levels.
- Maintain good posture and joint alignment to avoid injury.

What to Eat Before and After Strength Training

A light pre-workout snack (e.g., 100g fruit or unsweetened fruit smoothie) helps prevent hypoglycemia...

Who Should Avoid or Modify Strength Training?

Certain conditions may require caution or modification:

- Proliferative diabetic retinopathy
- Severe diabetic neuropathy or foot ulcers
- Chronic kidney disease (CKD Stage 4 or 5)
- Recent stroke or cardiovascular events

Final Word

Resistance training is not just for bodybuilders—it is medicine for your muscles, metabolism, and longevity. For Indian diabetics—especially those over 40—it's time to look beyond walking. Building muscle is not vanity; it's vitality.

Scientific References

1. Dunstan DW et al. High-intensity resistance training improves glycemic control in older patients with type 2 diabetes. Diabetes Care. 2002.

2. Sigal RJ et al. Aerobic exercise vs resistance training in type 2 diabetes. Ann Intern Med. 2007.
3. Church TS et al. Effects of aerobic and resistance training on hemoglobin A1c levels in patients with type 2 diabetes. JAMA. 2010.
4. American Diabetes Association. Standards of Medical Care in Diabetes—2024. Diabetes Care. 2024.
5. Colberg SR et al. Exercise and Type 2 Diabetes: ACSM and ADA Joint Position Statement. Diabetes Care. 2016.

CHAPTER 6

RUNNING AND DIABETES – STRIDE SMART FOR BETTER METABOLIC HEALTH

Pros and Cons of Running for Diabetes and Metabolic Health

☑ **Pros**

- Improves Insulin Sensitivity – enhances GLUT-4 activity in muscles, improving glucose uptake.
- Lowers Blood Glucose and HbA1c – shown to reduce fasting blood sugar and HbA1c.
- Enhances Cardiovascular Fitness – improves VO_2 max and reduces cardiac risks.
- Promotes Fat Loss, especially visceral fat, which worsens insulin resistance.
- Boosts Mitochondrial Health – improves metabolic flexibility.
- Reduces Stress – lowers cortisol and promotes endorphin release.

- Improves Lipid Profile – reduces triglycerides and inflammation.

⚠ Cons

- Risk of Hypoglycemia – especially in insulin or sulfonylurea users without proper planning.
- Foot Injuries – higher risk in those with diabetic neuropathy.
- Not Ideal in Retinopathy – risk of aggravating fragile retinal blood vessels.
- Joint Stress – particularly for overweight or older individuals.
- Glycemic Variability – blood sugar may spike or drop unpredictably post-run.
- Sustainability Issues – motivation, weather, and joint limitations may hinder long-term adherence.

Don't Just Run – Build: Why Protein and Strength Training Are Essential for Runners With Diabetes

Many individuals—especially in India—take up running as their primary or only form of exercise. While running is an excellent cardiovascular workout, doing it in isolation without adequate protein intake or resistance training can hinder long-term metabolic health, particularly in people with type 2 diabetes or prediabetes.

⚠ What Happens When You Only Run:

- Muscle Loss – Without resistance training and protein, runners may lose muscle mass, reducing insulin sensitivity.
- Injury Risk – Inadequate protein delays muscle recovery and increases joint stress.

- Plateaued Glucose Control – Cardio alone can lose its metabolic edge over time.
- Hormonal Imbalance – Excessive cardio may increase cortisol and decrease testosterone.

✅ What Smart Runners Do Differently:

- Eat Enough Protein – Aim for 1.0–1.2 g/kg/day from high-quality sources.
- Add Resistance Training Twice Weekly – Bodyweight exercises like squats and planks can suffice.
- Use Resistance Bands or Light Weights – Ideal for beginners or non-gym users.
- Balance Workouts – Combine 3 sessions of running with 2 strength sessions each week.

Final Word

Running helps you burn glucose, but muscle helps you manage it. Without protein and strength training, you're just running in circles.

Scientific References

1. Colberg SR et al. (2024). Exercise and Type 2 Diabetes: 2024 Update by the American Diabetes Association. Diabetes Care, 47(Suppl 1): S173–S191.
2. Bird SR et al. (2022). Effects of endurance training and resistance training on glycemic control in type 2 diabetes: A systematic review and meta-analysis. Sports Medicine, 52(3), 455–468.

3. Malin SK et al. (2021). Exercise as Medicine for Type 2 Diabetes: Prescribing the Right Dose. Current Sports Medicine Reports, 20(6), 287–294.

CHAPTER 7

THE PURPOSE-DRIVEN PATH TO REVERSING DIABETES

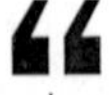

"Purpose is the most powerful prescription ever written—and it comes with no side effects."

– Unknown

◈ Introduction: More Than Willpower

Diabetes is not just a condition of the pancreas. It's often a reflection of lifestyle, stress, and emotional disconnection. Behind every lasting health transformation is not just a to-do list, but a deeply personal 'why.' When people reconnect with purpose, their physiology follows. Motivation is not found in lectures but in meaning.

◈ Science Behind Purpose and Health

◈ Turning Awareness into Action

For many, diabetes care starts as a reaction—following doctor's orders, counting steps, skipping sweets. But healing truly begins when action becomes self-directed and personally meaningful. People who find purpose in their choices often go further than those just trying to 'be compliant.' The shift from passive to purposeful care is often the real turning point.

Scientific research consistently shows that people with a strong sense of life purpose are healthier, live longer, and are less likely to develop chronic conditions, including Type 2 diabetes. A 2023 meta-analysis in Diabetes Care found that structured behavioral therapy based on personal goals significantly reduced HbA1c levels. Purpose-driven individuals tend to sleep better, eat more mindfully, and maintain better metabolic control.

◈ Rediscovering Meaning: Questions Worth Asking

- What excites you enough to wake up joyfully?
- Who or what do you want to be fully present for?
- What legacy would you like your health to enable?
- How does staying metabolically fit help you serve your deeper mission?

◈ Tools to Cultivate Inner Motivation

- Write a 'Why Statement' and keep it visible.
- Reflect daily on what you're grateful for and how your body helps you.
- Set identity-based goals: 'I am a strong, conscious person who makes healthy choices.'
- Avoid perfection—focus on direction.

– Build habits that align with values, not just numbers.

◈ Case Reflection

A 48-year-old man reversed his Type 2 diabetes not when his doctor increased his medication, but when his first grandson was born. He said, 'I want to live long enough to teach him cricket.' That single vision anchored his discipline more than any app ever could.

◈ Key Takeaways

– True healing begins with meaning.
– When the 'why' is strong, the 'how' becomes doable.
– Diabetes care must also be soul care.

References

1. Boyle PA et al. Purpose in life and incident diabetes in older adults. Psychosomatic Medicine. 2010.
2. Kim ES, Sun JK, Park N, et al. Purpose in life and reduced incidence of stroke in older adults. J Psychosom Res. 2013.
3. American Diabetes Association. Standards of Medical Care in Diabetes—2025.
4. Frankl V. Man's Search for Meaning. Beacon Press.
5. Mezuk B, et al. Depression and Type 2 Diabetes: A Bidirectional Association. Diabetes Care. 2020.

SECTION 5

DIABETES COMPANION CHAPTERS

CHAPTER 1

GROWING UP WITH SUGAR – DIABETES IN ADOLESCENTS AND TEENS

Introduction

Adolescence is a challenging phase on its own—add diabetes to the mix, and it becomes a rollercoaster. Teenagers face hormonal shifts, emotional highs and lows, peer pressure, and a desire for independence—all of which can affect blood sugar control.

This chapter explores the unique dynamics of managing diabetes during the teenage years, covering both Type 1 and rising cases of early-onset Type 2 diabetes.

1. **Rising Tide: Why More Teens Are Getting Diabetes**
   - Sedentary lifestyle, junk food, screen addiction, and obesity are driving early-onset Type 2 diabetes in Indian teens.
   - PCOS in girls, family history, and insulin resistance are key contributors.

- Type 1 diabetes continues to emerge in children under 18, requiring lifelong insulin therapy.

2. Puberty and Blood Sugar – A Turbulent Mix

- Hormonal changes during puberty increase insulin resistance.
- Teens may need more insulin or see higher sugar levels temporarily.
- Emotional stress and irregular sleep add to sugar fluctuations.

3. Teen Psychology: The Hidden Struggle

- Many teens feel different, frustrated, or rebellious about their diagnosis.
- Common issues:

* Skipping insulin doses
* Eating in secret
* Social withdrawal
* Mental health challenges (anxiety, depression)

- Family and peer support are critical. So is involving teens in their own care planning.

4. Early Type 2 – Not a Milder Form

- Teen-onset Type 2 progresses faster than adult-onset Type 2.
- Higher risk of early complications such as kidney disease, fatty liver, and retinopathy.
- Common in overweight or sedentary teens with a family history.

- Often misunderstood as 'milder'—but it is aggressive and requires urgent lifestyle change.

"MODY (Maturity-Onset Diabetes of the Young):"

- A genetic form of diabetes, often misdiagnosed as Type 1 or 2.
- Typically develops before age 25.
- Usually inherited; some types may not require insulin.
- Diagnosis is confirmed by genetic testing and family history.

"LADA (Latent Autoimmune Diabetes in Adults):"

- Sometimes seen in older teens or young adults.
- Autoimmune in origin, like Type 1, but with slower progression.
- Initially controlled by tablets, but later requires insulin.
- Often misdiagnosed as Type 2—antibody testing helps confirm.

5. Diet and Exercise for Teens

- Teens need real, non-preachy guidance. Focus on:
  Balanced meals with fiber, protein, and good fats
  Avoiding fruit juices, soda, bakery items, fried snacks
  Regular sports, dancing, or gym (not forced walks)
  Setting screen time limits without sounding like a lecture

6. Managing School and Social Life

- Inform school authorities discreetly about diabetes.
- Carry hypo snacks and water at all times.
- Teach teens how to manage sugars during exams, sports, outings.

- Encourage structured routines but allow flexibility for birthdays, trips, etc.

7. **Transition to Adult Care**

- As teens turn 18, they move from pediatric to adult care.
- They must learn to take charge—knowing their medications, lab targets, and when to seek help.
- Avoid over-parenting or complete detachment. Balance is key.

Success Story: Aayushi, 17 – From Frustrated to Empowered

Diagnosed with Type 1 at 13, Aayushi hated insulin and fought with her parents about food.

Through structured counseling and peer support:

- She joined a teen diabetes group.
- Learned carb counting.
- Now shares her journey on Instagram to help others.

Her HbA1c improved from 10.2% to 7.8% in 9 months.

Conclusion

Teenagers don't need perfection—they need "understanding, flexibility, and empowerment".

Managing diabetes in teens is less about control and more about building habits that will last a lifetime.

"Let teens be young—but also strong, smart, and sugar-aware."

References

1. Dabelea D, et al. Type 2 diabetes in youth: epidemiology and pathophysiology. Diabetes Care. 2014;37(2):402–408.
2. Shepherd M, Hattersley AT. 'Maturity-onset diabetes of the young' (MODY): Clinical features, diagnosis and management. Br J Diabetes Vasc Dis. 2004;4(1):13–20.
3. Naik RG, Brooks-Worrell BM, Palmer JP. Latent autoimmune diabetes in adults. J Clin Endocrinol Metab. 2009;94(12):4635–4644.
4. International Society for Pediatric and Adolescent Diabetes (ISPAD) Clinical Practice Consensus Guidelines 2022.

CHAPTER 2

METABOLIC KARMA – HOW CHILDHOOD HABITS SHAPE ADULT DIABETES

Introduction

Diabetes doesn't begin with blood sugar—it begins with habits. The seeds of metabolic disease are often sown in childhood, long before the first elevated glucose reading.

From poor diets and inactivity to chronic stress and screen addiction, early-life patterns silently shape how the body handles insulin, stores fat, and responds to inflammation. This chapter unpacks how these habits form the 'metabolic karma' of adult life.

1. The Childhood Origins of a Lifelong Disease

- Early onset of central obesity and fatty liver
- High-carb, low-protein diets in children
- Sugar-laden tiffin boxes, lack of vegetables and good fats

- Parents using food as a reward or emotional comfort

2. **Screen Time – The Silent Metabolic Poison**

   - Excessive screen use = less physical activity + worse sleep
   - Promotes mindless snacking and dopamine-driven junk cravings
   - Disrupts circadian rhythm and melatonin production
   - Studies show increased insulin resistance with >2 hrs/day of screen time in kids

3. **Sleep Debt in Children – A Hidden Hormonal Storm**

   - Late-night mobile use, academic stress, and social media reduce deep sleep
   - Sleep deprivation increases ghrelin (hunger hormone) and decreases leptin (satiety hormone)
   - Poor sleep is directly linked to childhood obesity and early insulin resistance

4. **Movement vs. Exercise – Reframing for Kids**

   - Children don't need gyms—they need movement:
     Outdoor play
     Sports
     Dance
     Martial arts
   - Structured routines like yoga or team games also boost discipline and emotional health

5. Gut Health and Ultra-Processed Foods

- Modern diets are low in fiber, fermented foods, and diversity
- Frequent antibiotics in early life damage the gut microbiome
- Gut health is now linked to insulin sensitivity, mood, and even learning ability

6. How Parents Can Reset the Cycle

- Focus on protein-rich breakfasts (eggs, paneer, sprouts)
- Limit screens to <1 hour/day (non-academic)
- Encourage family walks, tech-free dinners, and structured bedtimes
- Replace chips with nuts, juices with buttermilk or lemon water
- Talk about health—not weight—to build body positivity

Case Study: Rishi, 12 – A Turnaround Story

Rishi was a 12-year-old boy with obesity, dark neck patches, and borderline fasting insulin. He played no sport, loved chips, and slept past midnight daily.

- At his father's consultation, a metabolic reset was initiated:
  * Protein-first breakfasts
  * Screen limit to 60 mins/day
  * Family yoga and walks 3x/week
- In 6 months, he lost 4 kg, reversed insulin resistance, and joined his school's basketball team.

Conclusion

The metabolic health of a nation starts in its playgrounds, not ICUs. What children eat, how they move, and how they sleep determine their future risk for diabetes, heart disease, and more.

"Today's childhood habits are tomorrow's blood reports."

References

1. Narasimhan S, Weinstock RS. Youth-onset type 2 diabetes mellitus: lessons learned from the TODAY study. Mayo Clin Proc. 2014;89(6):806-816.
2. Hales CM, Carroll MD, Fryar CD, Ogden CL. Prevalence of obesity among children and adolescents: United States, trends 1963–1965 through 2015–2016. National Center for Health Statistics.

CHAPTER 3

DIABETES IN THE ELDERLY – BEYOND SUGAR, BEYOND PILLS

Introduction

India's aging population is living longer, but also living with more disease. Diabetes in older adults presents unique challenges that require a gentler, individualized approach. Rather than just managing glucose numbers, we must focus on preserving functionality, independence, and quality of life.

Why Elderly Diabetics Deserve Special Attention

With age, the body becomes more vulnerable to infections, falls, cognitive decline, and medication side effects. Diabetes increases these risks. Managing diabetes in the elderly requires a shift from 'tight control' to 'safe control'.

The Polypharmacy Trap

– Elderly patients often take 8–15 medications daily.

- Common drug classes: diabetes meds, antihypertensives, statins, PPIs, sedatives, painkillers.
- Risks include:
  Drug–drug interactions
  Hypoglycemia
  Falls and fractures
  Reduced kidney function
  Poor medication adherence

Hypoglycemia – The Hidden Danger

- Older adults often miss or misinterpret low sugar symptoms.
- Confusion, fainting, falls, and fatigue may be signs.
- Repeated lows can worsen memory and heart health.

Diabetes and the Brain

- High sugars are linked to cognitive decline and Alzheimer's disease.
- Memory loss may lead to skipped or double medication doses.
- Monitoring and simplifying regimens are essential.

Muscle Loss and Frailty

- Sarcopenia (muscle loss) is common in elderly diabetics.
- It worsens insulin resistance and increases fall risk.
- Solutions:
  * Adequate protein intake (1–1.2 g/kg ideal weight)
  * Strength exercises (resistance bands, sit-stands, wall pushups)

Tailoring Targets for the Elderly

In my clinical practice, I aim for safe and sustainable targets. Strict control increases hypoglycemia risk.

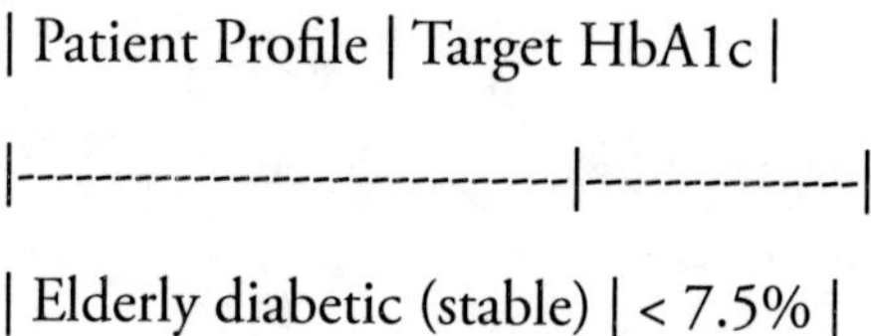

Patient Profile	Target HbA1c
Elderly diabetic (stable)	< 7.5%

More aggressive targets are not required unless strongly indicated.

What Works in My Clinical Practice

In my own practice, I focus on:

- Reducing pill burden by stopping unnecessary or marginally effective medications.
- Retaining low-dose metformin if tolerated.
- Improving protein nutrition.
- Ensuring adequate hydration, movement, and restful sleep.
- Educating families about recognizing low sugars and drug side effects.

Case Study: Mrs. Nirmala, 76 – From Tired to Thriving

Mrs. Nirmala, age 76, came with fatigue and two recent falls. She was on 9 medications including glimepiride and alprazolam.

- We simplified her regimen: stopped sulfonylurea, retained low-dose metformin.
- Focused on protein nutrition (70 g/day) and 15-minute walks.
- Outcome: No falls in 12 months, more alert and active.

Conclusion

Diabetes in the elderly is not about chasing numbers—it's about protecting dignity, independence, and safety.

Fewer medicines, thoughtful nutrition, gentle movement, and support systems matter far more than just sugar targets.

"In the elderly, safety is success."

References

1. American Diabetes Association. Older Adults: Standards of Medical Care in Diabetes—2024. Diabetes Care. 2024;47(Suppl 1):S229–S239.
2. Sinclair AJ, et al. Managing older people with type 2 diabetes: Global guideline. International Diabetes Federation. 2014.
3. Morley JE, et al. Frailty consensus: a call to action. J Am Med Dir Assoc. 2013;14(6):392–397.
4. Lipska KJ, et al. Potential overtreatment of diabetes mellitus in older adults with tight glycemic control. JAMA Intern Med. 2015;175(3):356–362.

CHAPTER 4

SUGAR IN THE WOMB – THE HIDDEN CRISIS OF GESTATIONAL DIABETES

Gestational Diabetes Mellitus (GDM) is a common but often underrecognized complication during pregnancy, especially in India. This condition not only affects maternal health but also has long-lasting consequences for the offspring.

Interesting Facts About Gestational Diabetes

🌍 India has one of the highest burdens of gestational diabetes in the world.

👶 Babies born to mothers with uncontrolled GDM are at higher risk of childhood obesity and diabetes.

📈 Nearly 50–60% of Indian women with GDM will go on to develop Type 2 diabetes within 5–10 years.

💡 Women who breastfeed after GDM have a lower risk of future diabetes.

🥗 Low glycemic index (GI) diets not only reduce sugar spikes but also lower insulin requirements in pregnancy.

📚 Guidelines for Diagnosing GDM

- The American Diabetes Association (ADA, 2025) and WHO recommend screening all pregnant women between 24–28 weeks.
- In India, the DIPSI (Diabetes in Pregnancy Study Group India) recommends a one-step test using 75g oral glucose irrespective of fasting state.
- GDM is diagnosed if 2-hour plasma glucose ≥ 140 mg/dL after a 75g glucose load.
- For high-risk women (obesity, PCOS, history of GDM), early screening in the first trimester is advised.

◈ Medical Nutrition Therapy (MNT): The Foundation of GDM Management

- MNT involves individualized meal planning by a trained dietician based on weight, gestational age, and glycemic goals.
- ADA 2025 recommends 3 small-to-moderate meals and 2–4 snacks to maintain glucose stability.
- Carbohydrates should make up 35–45% of total calories, focusing on low glycemic index sources.
- Meals should include a balance of protein (paneer, dal, tofu, eggs), healthy fats (nuts, seeds, oils), and vegetables.
- Regular blood glucose monitoring (fasting and postprandial) is essential to evaluate dietary adequacy.
- MNT alone is effective in 70–85% of cases, reducing the need for pharmacotherapy.

Monitoring and Management of Gestational Diabetes

- Blood sugar levels must be checked frequently using a glucometer.
- Recommended monitoring includes: Fasting blood sugar, 1 or 2 hours post-meal sugar levels.
- Target blood glucose levels: Fasting: <95 mg/dL, 1-hour postprandial: <140 mg/dL, 2-hour postprandial: <120 mg/dL.
- Continuous Glucose Monitoring (CGM) can be considered in select cases for real-time tracking, especially in insulin-requiring patients.
- CGMs offer advantages like trend analysis, alerts for hypo/hyperglycemia, and improved glycemic control with less finger pricking.

Treatment and Pharmacologic Management

- Diet and lifestyle are first-line treatment for GDM.
- If blood sugars remain uncontrolled despite MNT, insulin therapy is the treatment of choice.
- Insulin does not harm the baby and is safe during pregnancy.
- Oral medications like metformin may be considered in specific cases under supervision.
- Regular follow-up with healthcare professionals ensures timely adjustments to therapy.

Common Dietary Myths to Avoid

Indian Pregnancy Myth	Why It's Problematic
"Eat for two"	Leads to overeating, excessive weight gain, sugar spikes

"All fruits are safe during pregnancy"	High-fructose fruits (like mango, grapes) spike sugars
"Fruit juices and smoothies are healthy"	Lack of fiber, causes rapid blood sugar elevations
"No need to control carbs in home food"	Refined carbs in rotis, rice, poha, etc., add up quickly

Quick Recap

- Gestational Diabetes affects 1 in 5 Indian pregnancies and often goes unnoticed.
- Early screening (24–28 weeks) is essential and even earlier for high-risk women.
- Dietary management with a low-GI, protein-rich plan is the first-line treatment.
- Monitoring sugar levels using a glucometer or CGM is vital for the mother and baby's health.
- Medical nutrition therapy (MNT) alone can manage GDM in up to 85% of cases.
- Insulin is safe in pregnancy; metformin may be used in specific situations.

References

1. American Diabetes Association. Standards of Care in Diabetes—2025. Diabetes Care. 2025;48(Suppl 1):S144-S150.

2. World Health Organization. Diagnostic criteria and classification of hyperglycaemia first detected in pregnancy. Geneva: WHO; 2023.
3. Diabetes in Pregnancy Study Group India (DIPSI) Guidelines. Indian J Endocrinol Metab. 2023;27(1):38-45.
4. Jovanovic L. Medical management of pregnancy complicated by diabetes. Clinical Diabetes. 2024.
5. International Diabetes Federation. IDF Diabetes Atlas 2024, 11th edition.

CHAPTER 5

YOUR LIVER KNOWS – FATTY LIVER AND DIABETES: TWO SIDES OF THE SAME COIN

You might not feel it, but your liver is quietly shaping your metabolic destiny. Metabolic Dysfunction-Associated Fatty Liver Disease (MAFLD), formerly known as NAFLD, is becoming a silent epidemic in India—especially among those with prediabetes or Type 2 diabetes. It's a metabolic warning sign. This chapter explores how fatty liver and diabetes are deeply interconnected, and how fixing one often improves the other.

🔄 Did You Know?

What was once called NAFLD (Non-Alcoholic Fatty Liver Disease) is now globally redefined as MAFLD (Metabolic Dysfunction-Associated Fatty Liver Disease). This reflects the true root cause—metabolic dysfunction—not alcohol. The term MAFLD was officially adopted by global medical bodies starting in 2023 to more accurately represent patients with obesity, insulin resistance, or Type 2 diabetes.

🩺 What Is MAFLD?

MAFLD refers to fat accumulation in liver cells in people who consume little or no alcohol. It ranges from simple steatosis to inflammation and fibrosis, formerly called NASH (Non-Alcoholic Steatohepatitis).

📌 Diagnostic Criteria for MAFLD

MAFLD is diagnosed when there is liver fat (on imaging or biopsy) and one of the following:

- Type 2 diabetes or prediabetes
- Overweight or obesity (BMI > 23 for South Asians)
- At least two metabolic risk factors (e.g., low HDL, high triglycerides, high waist circumference, raised CRP)

📊 The Growing Burden in India

- Over 30–40% of urban Indians have MAFLD
- Seen in 60–70% of those with diabetes
- Many lean individuals also develop MAFLD due to poor diet and genetics

🔗 How Fatty Liver is Linked to Diabetes

- Insulin resistance disrupts sugar metabolism
- Liver releases excess glucose
- Lipotoxicity and inflammation accelerate metabolic decline
- Up to 70% of people with diabetes have fatty liver
- MAFLD predicts diabetes even in lean individuals

How Reversing Fatty Liver Improves Diabetes—and Vice Versa

- Losing just 5–10% weight reduces liver fat
- Improves fasting sugars and HbA1c
- Reduces medication need
- Good glycemic control slows liver fibrosis

Think of it as a two-way street: Heal the liver to control sugar. Control the sugar to heal the liver.

References

1. Eslam M, Sanyal AJ, George J. MAFLD: A Consensus-Driven Proposed Nomenclature. Gastroenterology. 2020.
2. Chalasani N, Younossi Z, Lavine JE, et al. AASLD Guidelines for NAFLD. Hepatology. 2018.
3. Younossi ZM, et al. Global Epidemiology of NAFLD. Hepatology. 2016.
4. Bril F, Cusi K. Management of NAFLD in Type 2 Diabetes. Diabetes Care. 2017.
5. Kalra S, Unnikrishnan AG. MAFLD and Diabetes. Indian J Endocrinol Metab. 2020.
6. Armstrong MJ, et al. Liraglutide in NASH: LEAN Study. Lancet. 2016.

CHAPTER 6

THE GUT CONNECTION – HOW YOUR MICROBIOME SHAPES BLOOD SUGAR AND METABOLISM

Your gut is more than just a digestive tract — it's a complex ecosystem made up of trillions of microbes that can influence nearly every aspect of health, including blood sugar levels and metabolic function. Recent research has uncovered a strong link between gut health and the risk of developing Type 2 Diabetes.

What is the Gut Microbiome?

The gut microbiome is the community of bacteria, fungi, viruses, and other microorganisms that live in our intestines. These microbes help digest food, produce vitamins, and regulate immune responses. More recently, they have been found to affect insulin sensitivity and inflammation.

⚠ Gut Dysbiosis: A Hidden Trigger for Diabetes

Gut dysbiosis — an imbalance of good and bad microbes — has been observed in people with Type 2 Diabetes. Key patterns include:

- Reduced diversity of gut bacteria
- Increased levels of harmful endotoxins
- Elevated gut permeability ('leaky gut') that promotes chronic inflammation

These changes interfere with insulin signaling and can increase blood sugar levels over time.

🔬 Microbiome–Blood Sugar Axis: What We Know

- Certain bacteria (e.g., Akkermansia muciniphila, Bifidobacteria) have been associated with better glucose control.
- An unhealthy gut can increase production of lipopolysaccharides (LPS), which trigger insulin resistance.
- The gut also influences the release of hormones like GLP-1, which play a crucial role in glucose regulation.

🌿 How to Nurture Your Gut for Blood Sugar Stability

- Include more fermented foods like curd, kefir, idli, dosa, and kanji.
- Eat a fiber-rich diet — whole vegetables, greens, and seeds like flax or chia.
- Avoid excessive antibiotics and painkillers unless medically necessary.

- Cut down on ultra-processed foods that feed harmful gut bacteria.
- Consider a high-quality probiotic supplement (under medical advice).
- Practice mindful eating and chew thoroughly — digestion begins in the mouth.

🔮 What the Future Holds

Scientists are working on developing precision-based microbiome therapies for diabetes—including tailored probiotics, microbiota transplants, and even AI-based gut profiling. These innovations may redefine how we prevent and treat metabolic disorders in the near future.

🔁 Quick Recap

- The gut microbiome is a vast ecosystem of microbes that significantly impact blood sugar and metabolism.
- Imbalance in gut bacteria (dysbiosis) is linked to insulin resistance and Type 2 Diabetes.
- Key protective gut bacteria like Akkermansia and Bifidobacteria support better glucose control.
- Improving gut health through fermented foods, fiber, and probiotics may aid in diabetes management.
- Future treatments may involve personalized microbiome therapies to prevent and reverse diabetes.

References

1. Gurung M, et al. Role of gut microbiota in type 2 diabetes pathophysiology. EBioMedicine. 2020;51:102590.
2. Zhao L, et al. Gut bacteria selectively promoted by dietary fibers alleviate type 2 diabetes. Science. 2018;359(6380):1151–1156.
3. Thaiss CA, et al. Microbiome dynamics in diabetes and metabolic disease. Cell Metab. 2016;24(4):572–582.
4. Indian Journal of Endocrinology and Metabolism. Gut microbiota and metabolic disorders: An Indian perspective. IJEM. 2023.
5. NIH Human Microbiome Project. U.S. Department of Health and Human Services, 2024.

CHAPTER 7

THE NEW FAT BURNERS – GAME-CHANGING DRUGS TRANSFORMING DIABETES AND WEIGHT LOSS

> "What if your diabetes medication could also help you lose 15 to 20 kilos—and protect your heart at the same time?"

It sounds too good to be true—but it's not. A new generation of medications is changing how we approach both diabetes and obesity—two conditions that are tightly linked by insulin resistance, inflammation, and metabolic dysfunction. These drugs don't just lower blood sugar—they help shed significant weight, improve cholesterol, and reduce cardiovascular risk. Welcome to the era of incretin-based therapies.

The Metabolic Breakthrough: What Are These Drugs?

Most of these novel drugs are based on a class called GLP-1 receptor agonists. Some also target GIP and glucagon receptors—hence called dual or triple agonists.

They mimic or enhance the action of gut hormones called incretins that:
- Increase insulin secretion (only when needed)
- Reduce glucagon (the hormone that raises blood sugar)
- Slow down gastric emptying (so you feel full longer)
- Suppress appetite via the brain

These actions together lower blood sugar and reduce hunger—creating a powerful dual impact.

Meet the Superstars: A New Lineup of Drugs

1. **Semaglutide (Ozempic, Wegovy, Rybelsus)**

- Weekly injectable (Ozempic, Wegovy) or daily oral tablet (Rybelsus)
- FDA-approved for Type 2 diabetes (Ozempic) and obesity (Wegovy)
- In clinical trials, people lost up to 15% of their body weight
- Improves HbA1c, reduces risk of cardiovascular events
- In India: Ozempic and Rybelsus are available; Wegovy is expected soon

Backed by Trials:
- STEP trials (for obesity)
- SUSTAIN trials (for diabetes)

2. Tirzepatide (Mounjaro)

- Weekly injection
- Dual GIP + GLP-1 receptor agonist
- Promotes 20%+ weight loss in clinical trials—approaching results seen with bariatric surgery
- Now officially available in India as of March 2025, following approval by the CDSCO
- Can be prescribed for both Type 2 diabetes and obesity

Backed by Trials:

- SURMOUNT and SURPASS trials
- HbA1c reductions up to 2.5%, along with significant improvements in body weight, blood pressure, and lipid profile

3. Liraglutide (Victoza, Saxenda)

- Older GLP-1 agonist; daily injection
- Saxenda: approved for weight loss
- Victoza: approved for diabetes
- Moderate weight loss (~6–8%)
- Still used in India, especially when newer agents are not affordable

4. Coming Soon: Retatrutide

- Triple action on GLP-1, GIP, and glucagon receptors
- In Phase 2 trials, participants lost over 25% of their body weight
- May become the most powerful non-surgical tool for obesity and diabetes yet

Why This Matters: Weight Loss = Better Sugar Control

Even a 5% reduction in body weight improves:

- Insulin sensitivity
- HbA1c levels
- Lipid profiles
- Liver fat (reduced NAFLD)
- Blood pressure
- Cardiovascular risk

With drugs like semaglutide and tirzepatide, 15–20% weight loss is achievable—often without hypoglycemia or hunger pangs.

Side Effects and Cautions

Common:

- Nausea
- Vomiting
- Constipation
- Loss of appetite

Rare but important:

- Pancreatitis (rare, but a theoretical risk)
- Gallstones (with rapid weight loss)
- Slight increase in heart rate
- Thyroid C-cell tumors (in rodents, not confirmed in humans)

Most side effects improve with time or dose adjustment.

Who Are These Drugs For?

Ideal candidates:

- Type 2 diabetics with BMI >27
- Those with insulin resistance or fatty liver
- People at high cardiovascular risk
- Individuals struggling to lose weight despite lifestyle changes

These are prescription-only medications and must be started under medical supervision, especially if other diabetes medications are being used simultaneously.

The Dark Side: Misuse, Myths, and Medical Ethics

The success of these medications has led to rampant off-label use, especially among individuals:

- Without diabetes
- With only mild overweight
- Seeking rapid weight loss for cosmetic or social media appeal

Misuse is a real concern. There's growing misuse of Mounjaro and Ozempic among celebrities, influencers, and the public purely for aesthetics—not for medical necessity. This has caused:

- Global shortages for diabetic patients
- Increased risk of side effects in unsupervised use
- Public misconception that these are miracle weight-loss drugs

Yet, one fact remains: Reducing excess body fat—especially visceral fat—dramatically improves insulin sensitivity. Even in non-diabetics, fat loss from GLP-1 or dual agonists can:

- Lower fasting insulin

- Reduce HOMA-IR
- Decrease inflammation
- Delay or prevent the onset of Type 2 diabetes

But the method and context matter. Reckless or aesthetic-only use undermines their purpose and risks side effects, dependency, and public distrust.

The Mindset Shift: This Is Not a Shortcut

These drugs must be used:

- Under medical supervision
- As part of a comprehensive lifestyle plan
- With nutritional and behavioral support to maintain long-term results

They are not weight-loss hacks. They are metabolic reset tools.

Indian Scenario: Cost, Access, and Awareness

In India:

- Ozempic and Rybelsus are already available
- Mounjaro (tirzepatide) launched in March 2025
- Insurance rarely covers weight-loss medications
- Many doctors hesitate to prescribe due to limited awareness or cost concerns

This chapter aims to bridge that gap and empower both patients and healthcare professionals.

The Future Is Bright (and Injectable...for Now)

Upcoming innovations:

– Oral versions of GLP-1 + GIP drugs
– Longer-acting injectables (monthly dosing)
– Personalized medicine based on your metabolic profile

These drugs are also being studied for:

– PCOS
– NAFLD
– Addiction
– Alzheimer's disease

FAQs

Q: Can I stop my insulin or other medications after starting this?

→ Possibly, but only under supervision.

Q: Are these drugs safe long term?

→ Trials up to 5 years show excellent results with cardiovascular benefits. Long-term studies are ongoing.

Q: Will I regain the weight if I stop?

→ Weight regain is likely unless you continue lifestyle changes. These drugs "buy you time" to make deeper habit changes.

Takeaway

"Obesity is not a failure of willpower. It's a hormonal imbalance. And now, we have tools to help rebalance it."

For decades, diabetes management was about lowering sugar. Now, it's about reversing the root causes—insulin resistance, excess fat, and inflammation.

These new medications aren't magic. But in the hands of informed doctors and committed patients, they can be transformational.

References

1. Wilding JP, et al. N Engl J Med, 2021; 384:989–1002. (STEP 1 Trial)
2. Frias JP, et al. N Engl J Med, 2021; 385:503–515. (SURPASS trials)
3. Rubino D, et al. Lancet, 2021; 397:971–984. (SUSTAIN trial data)
4. American Diabetes Association. Standards of Medical Care in Diabetes – 2025.
5. Jastreboff AM et al. New England Journal of Medicine, 2023. (Retatrutide Phase 2 trial)

CHAPTER 8

MONITORING SUGARS IN THE DIGITAL AGE – BEYOND FINGER PRICKS

"What gets measured gets managed." This age-old wisdom has never been more relevant than in diabetes care today. With technology evolving faster than ever, the way we monitor blood sugars has undergone a digital revolution—from painful finger pricks to real-time data streams on our phones.

In this chapter, we explore the emerging tools of the digital age, how they're transforming patient engagement, and how to use them wisely, not obsessively.

1. The Traditional Monitoring: Still Relevant, But Limited

- Self-Monitoring of Blood Glucose (SMBG):
- Involves finger-stick glucose testing using a glucometer.
- Common readings include fasting, post-meal, and bedtime sugars.
- Affordable, simple, and still the mainstay for many.
- Limitations:
- Provides only snapshot data.

- Painful for some, leading to poor adherence.
- Misses trends like nocturnal hypoglycemia or postprandial spikes.

2. **The Game-Changer: Continuous Glucose Monitoring (CGM)**

   - A small sensor inserted under the skin measures glucose in interstitial fluid every few minutes.
   - Types of CGMs:
   - Professional (retrospective)
   - Real-time CGM (RT-CGM)
   - Flash Glucose Monitoring (FGM)
   - Key Metrics:
   - Time in Range (TIR)
   - Time Below Range (TBR)
   - Glycemic Variability
   - Glucose Management Indicator (GMI)

3. **Benefits of CGM: More Than Just Numbers**

   - Improved glycemic control
   - Real-time feedback encourages behavior change
   - Empowers patients
   - Reduces HbA1c even in patients with long-standing type 2 diabetes

4. **Smart Integration: Apps, Alerts, and AI**

   - Apps like LibreLink, Dexcom G7, Sugarmate, and mySugr

- Cloud-based sharing with doctors
- AI-driven insights to predict trends and warn of hypoglycemia

5. Challenges in the Indian Context

- Cost remains a barrier
- Awareness is still low
- Data overload can lead to anxiety
- Over-reliance on tech without lifestyle change

6. Who Should Use CGM in India? (2025 Perspective)

- Patients on multiple insulin injections or insulin pumps
- Those with hypoglycemia unawareness
- Pregnant women with type 1 or gestational diabetes
- Motivated type 2 diabetics
- Athletes or fitness enthusiasts with diabetes

7. Wearables and Smartwatches – Are They Accurate?

- Non-invasive sensors currently lack accuracy
- Some watches integrate with CGMs for display only
- Future may bring non-invasive glucose sensing

8. The Smart Way to Use CGM

Do This:

- Use TIR, GMI, and variability data
- Share reports with your doctor
- Pair CGM insights with logs
- Take breaks if CGM fatigue sets in

Avoid This:
- Obsessing over every up-and-down
- Making random changes
- Using CGM without action
- Wearing 24x7 without rest

9. A Note on HbA1c in the Digital Era

- HbA1c is still the gold standard
- Misses fluctuations and hypoglycemia risks
- Use HbA1c + CGM + patient behavior together

10. The Future of Digital Diabetes Monitoring

- Closed-loop systems
- Predictive analytics
- Gamification
- Insurance-linked incentives in India

Final Word

The digital age offers powerful tools—but the goal remains the same: Know your numbers, understand your body, and act with awareness. Whether you use a basic glucometer or the latest CGM, what matters is how well you use that data to steer your habits, not just your medications.

References

1. Battelino T, et al. Clinical Targets for Continuous Glucose Monitoring Data Interpretation: Diabetes Care. 2019.

2. Beck RW, et al. Effect of CGM on Glycemic Control in Adults With Type 2 Diabetes Using Basal Insulin. JAMA. 2017.
3. Aleppo G, et al. Benefits of Real-Time CGM in Type 2 Diabetes: Diabetes Technol Ther. 2021.
4. Shah VN, et al. Use of CGM in Developing Countries: Indian J Endocrinol Metab. 2020.

CHAPTER 9

THE FESTIVAL SURVIVAL GUIDE – ENJOY SWEETS WITHOUT SPIKING

Introduction

In India, festivals are sacred, vibrant, and sugar-laden. From Diwali to Eid, Christmas to birthdays, food is the love language of celebration. But for people with diabetes, these occasions can trigger anxiety or dangerous sugar spikes. This guide helps you enjoy festivals without inviting metabolic chaos.

Why Festivals Are a Sugar Minefield

– Overload of sweets, snacks, fried items
– Peer pressure and emotional eating
– Skipped meals followed by feasting
– Lack of activity or sleep

Mindset First: Plan, Don't Panic

You don't need perfection—just intention.
– Don't skip meals; eat light, fiber-rich foods earlier

– Choose one indulgence in advance
– Prioritize mindful eating over restriction

Enjoying Indian Sweets: The Smart Way

✅ Better Choices:

– Homemade low-carb sweets with almond flour, stevia
– Dry fruits with nuts (e.g., dates + walnuts)
– Traditional sweets in small portions post-meal

⚠ Watch Out For:

– High GI sweets like rasgulla, kaju katli
– Misleading sugar-free labels
– 'Diabetic sweets' from commercial shops

The One-Plate Festival Rule

– Half plate: vegetables/salad
– 1/4th plate: protein (paneer, dal, meat)
– 1/4th plate: carbs or sweets
– End with curd, buttermilk, or warm cinnamon water

Post-Meal Rituals That Reduce Sugar Spikes

– 15-minute walk post-meal
– Herbal tea with cinnamon or methi
– Seated relaxation to lower cortisol

Festive Sleep and Stress Tips

– Prioritize sleep before/after events
– Say no to food pushers politely
– Try deep breathing to manage stress

Recipes & Ideas for Diabetic-Friendly Festive Treats

1. Almond flour barfi with cardamom
2. Coconut laddoos with stevia & flaxseed
3. Paneer kheer with nut milk & chia
4. Baked methi mathri (almond base)
5. Steamed dhokla with grated carrot

Success Snapshot: Mrs. Nalini, 60 – Diwali Without Damage

Mrs. Nalini used to gain 2–3 kg every Diwali with sugar spikes. With Satva Clinic guidance:

- One laddoo/day post-lunch
- Higher protein meals
- Daily 20-min walks
- Homemade almond kheer

This Diwali: No weight gain, stable sugars, and no guilt.

Festivals Are For Joy, Not Guilt

Enjoy food, family, and traditions with awareness. You're not avoiding life—you're upgrading it.

"When you celebrate with wisdom, every sweet moment becomes a healthy memory."

CHAPTER 10

DIABETIC TRAVEL HACKS – STAYING ON TRACK AWAY FROM HOME

Introduction

Travel is one of life's greatest joys—but for people with diabetes, it can be a metabolic minefield. Changing time zones, unusual foods, missed meals, delayed medications, and lack of movement can wreak havoc on blood sugar levels.

But with some planning and practical tools, you can explore the world—or your hometown—without compromising your health.

1. Before You Go: Pre-Travel Checklist

- Get a medical review if you're traveling for more than a few days.
- Carry extra medications, prescriptions, glucometer strips, insulin pens, syringes, and alcohol swabs.
- Take copies of recent lab results and your doctor's note (especially for flights).

- If insulin-dependent, carry snacks for hypoglycemia and a printed hypo management card.

2. **Packing Like a Pro: Essentials for Every Diabetic**

   - Glucometer and strips in carry-on luggage
   - CGM sensors (if applicable)
   - Healthy snacks: almonds, peanuts, roasted chana, protein bars (no added sugar)
   - Hydration: Reusable water bottle
   - Oral rehydration salts for stomach upsets
   - Cold packs for insulin if traveling in hot weather

3. **Air Travel: Beat the Cabin Carb Trap**

   - Inform the airline of your diabetes while booking (diabetic meals may be available)
   - Avoid airline juices, breads, and sweets
   - Eat your own low-carb snack before boarding
   - Walk down the aisle every 2 hours to reduce insulin resistance and prevent clots
   - Adjust medication timing if crossing time zones—consult your doctor before long flights

4. **Trains, Road Trips & Bus Travel**

   - Indian trains often serve high-carb food—carry your own eggs, paneer cubes, roasted seeds, boiled peanuts, or methi parathas
   - On road trips, stop for walks every 2–3 hours
   - Avoid sugary drinks and fried snacks at stations or dhabas

- Always carry dry fruits and nut bars as a fallback

5. Hotel Hacks for Diabetics

- Book hotels with a mini-fridge or access to basic kitchenware
- Order protein-focused meals: grilled paneer, omelettes, boiled eggs, grilled chicken, sautéed vegetables
- Skip buffet excesses. Use the 'one-plate rule' with portion control
- Stay hydrated—hotel air conditioning can dehydrate silently

6. Exercise on the Go

- Walk the airport terminal before boarding
- Do 15-minute walks post meals, even in hotel corridors
- Use resistance bands or bodyweight workouts in your room
- Walking tours are better than vehicle tours for sugar control

7. Sick Day Rules While Traveling

- Monitor sugars more frequently
- Do not skip insulin or OHA even if the appetite is low
- Stick to small, frequent meals
- Stay hydrated with ORS or salted lemon water if vomiting/ loose stools occur
- Seek local medical help early if high sugars persist

8. Success Story: Mr. Krishnan, 64 – Himalayan Trekker with Diabetes

Mr. Krishnan, with Type 2 diabetes, went on a 7-day Himalayan trek after working with Satva Clinic:

- Carried roasted seeds, protein pouches, and boiled eggs
- Took glucose tabs for safety
- Kept a fixed walking and meal routine

His sugars remained stable throughout, and he returned healthier than before.

Conclusion

Diabetes shouldn't keep you home—it should teach you how to travel smart. With foresight, preparation, and a few hacks, you can explore the world while keeping your sugars in check.

"When you carry your health habits with you, no destination is off-limits."

References

1. American Diabetes Association. Diabetes and Travel. Diabetes Care. 2024;47(Supplement_1):S234-S236.
2. Bonora BM, Avogaro A, Fadini GP. Management of diabetes during travel. Endocrine. 2020;67(1):15–24.
3. Diabetes UK. Travel and holidays: Tips for managing diabetes on the go. Accessed May 2025. https://www.diabetes.org.uk/guide-to-diabetes/life-with-diabetes/travel

CHAPTER 11

DIABETES AND COGNITIVE DECLINE – THE FORGOTTEN LINK

Diabetes is often associated with blood sugar, feet, eyes, and heart, but what about the brain? Emerging research reveals a powerful and often overlooked connection between diabetes and cognitive function. In fact, poorly controlled diabetes may accelerate memory loss, brain fog, and even dementia. This chapter explores how and why this happens, and what you can do to protect your brain.

1. The Brain on Sugar – What Happens?

- The brain depends on a steady supply of glucose, but too much or too little is harmful.
- High blood sugar damages small vessels that nourish brain cells (microvascular damage).
- Insulin is not just for the body—it also regulates brain signaling, mood, and memory.

– Chronic hyperglycemia leads to inflammation, oxidative stress, and faster cognitive aging.

2. **Type 3 Diabetes – A New Name for Alzheimer's?**

   – Some researchers refer to Alzheimer's disease as "Type 3 Diabetes."
   – Studies show insulin resistance in the brain can impair learning and memory.
   – Beta-amyloid plaques and tau proteins are worsened by poor metabolic control.
   – People with type 2 diabetes have a 1.5 to 2x increased risk of developing dementia.

3. **Early Signs of Cognitive Trouble in Diabetes**

   – Forgetfulness, losing track of appointments or conversations.
   – Difficulty focusing or multitasking.
   – Reduced problem-solving or planning ability.
   – Mood changes, anxiety, or depressive symptoms.
   – Slower processing speed or decision-making.

4. **Who is Most at Risk?**

   – Long-standing diabetes (>10 years).
   – Frequent hypoglycemia episodes.
   – Poor HbA1c control over time (>8.5%).
   – Elderly individuals, especially those above 65.
   – People with co-existing high blood pressure, cholesterol, or stroke history.

5. How to Protect Your Brain – 7 Smart Strategies

- Keep blood sugars in target range—avoid highs *and* lows.
- Prioritize deep, restful sleep (7–8 hours).
- Engage in physical activity—especially strength and balance training.
- Eat brain-supportive foods (omega-3s, antioxidants, polyphenols).
- Stimulate the mind—read, play strategy games, learn new skills.
- Practice stress reduction—yoga, mindfulness, breathing.
- Limit processed carbs and trans fats—fuel your brain with whole foods.

6. Special Considerations in the Elderly

- Avoid tight sugar control in frail seniors to reduce hypoglycemia risk.
- Screen annually for memory and cognitive function in older diabetics.
- Involve caregivers in meal planning, medication reminders, and mental stimulation.
- Watch for subtle signs of decline—early intervention matters.

Final Word

Diabetes doesn't just affect your blood sugar—it affects your brain. By keeping your sugars steady, moving your body, sleeping well, and nourishing your mind, you can guard against cognitive decline and stay sharp for life. Remember, a healthy brain is the best reward for healthy blood sugar.

References

1. Biessels GJ, et al. Risk of dementia in diabetes mellitus: a systematic review. Lancet Neurol. 2006.
2. Arnold SE, et al. Brain insulin resistance in type 2 diabetes and Alzheimer's disease. J Clin Invest. 2018.
3. Rouch L, et al. Diabetes, cognitive impairment and dementia: systematic review and meta-analysis. J Alzheimers Dis. 2021.
4. Craft S. Insulin resistance and Alzheimer's disease pathogenesis: potential mechanisms. Curr Alzheimer Res. 2007.

CHAPTER 12

SUGAR, CELLS, AND CANCER – WHAT EVERY DIABETIC SHOULD KNOW

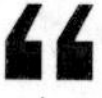

"Cancer feeds on sugar – but the story doesn't end there."

The Hidden Link We Don't Talk About

When we think of diabetes complications, we list heart attacks, kidney failure, eye disease. But there's a rising, quieter concern: Cancer.

Emerging research over the past decade has revealed something unsettling—people with type 2 diabetes have a higher risk of developing certain types of cancer.

Why? It's not just sugar. It's insulin, and how it acts like a growth hormone in overdrive.

What's the Link Between Diabetes and Cancer?

Diabetes, especially when uncontrolled, leads to:

- High insulin levels (hyperinsulinemia)
- Chronic inflammation
- Oxidative stress
- Visceral fat accumulation

These four together create an environment where cancer cells can grow, multiply, and survive longer.

Insulin is not just a sugar-regulating hormone, but also a powerful growth stimulator.

Which Cancers Are More Common in Diabetics?

Cancer Type	Relative Risk Increase
Liver cancer	2–3x
Pancreatic cancer	1.8–2x
Endometrial cancer	1.8x
Colorectal cancer	1.3–1.5x
Breast cancer (postmenopausal women)	1.2–1.3x
Bladder cancer	~1.2x

Why Insulin, Not Just Sugar, Is the Culprit

It's a common myth that sugar directly feeds cancer. What's truer is that cancer cells have a higher demand for glucose, and when insulin levels are high, the body is constantly in storage and growth mode—the very environment that helps precancerous cells grow unchecked.

What About Medications Like Metformin?

Interestingly, metformin, a commonly used diabetes drug, has shown anti-cancer effects in many observational studies. It:

- Lowers insulin levels
- Inhibits mTOR pathways
- Reduces cellular oxidative stress

Patients on metformin appear to have lower cancer incidence and mortality than those on insulin or sulfonylureas.

What Can You Do to Reduce Risk?

Even if you have diabetes, you can cut your cancer risk substantially with these steps:

☑ Control insulin resistance:
- Prioritize low glycemic foods
- Avoid frequent snacking
- Incorporate intermittent fasting

☑ Reduce visceral fat:
- Target waist circumference, not just weight
- Include resistance training and walking

☑ Use anti-inflammatory food choices:
- Turmeric, green tea, berries, cruciferous vegetables

☑ Avoid ultra-processed foods and seed oils

☑ Screen for cancer appropriately

Final Thought

Diabetes doesn't just raise your sugar. It alters your internal environment—your hormones, your inflammation levels, your body's ability to protect against rogue cells.

In this metabolic storm, cancer finds a fertile ground. But you can choose differently.

You can shift your body from a growth-promoting to a healing-promoting state—by lowering insulin, calming inflammation, and feeding your body with real, protective food.

Let your kitchen be your first line of defense.

Suggested References

1. Giovannucci E, et al. Diabetes and cancer: a consensus report. CA Cancer J Clin. 2010;60(4):207–221.
2. Tsilidis KK, et al. Type 2 diabetes and cancer: umbrella review of meta-analyses. BMJ. 2015;350:g7607.
3. Anisimov VN. Metformin: Do we finally have an anti-aging drug? Cell Cycle. 2013;12(22):3483–3489.
4. Dankner R, et al. Diabetes, glucose, insulin, and cancer. Lancet Oncol. 2016;17(10):e490–e505.
5. Indian Council of Medical Research (ICMR) – Cancer & Metabolic Disease Reports, 2023.

CHAPTER 13

THE SWEET DECEPTION – ARE DIET DRINKS REALLY SAFE FOR DIABETICS?

Walk down any supermarket aisle in India today, and you'll see a growing trend—people reaching not for regular Coke or Pepsi, but for their sleeker, zero-calorie cousins: Coke Zero, Diet Pepsi, Thumbs Up Light, or 7UP Free. The labels scream "zero sugar" and "no calories," promising guilt-free indulgence. For many living with diabetes, these drinks feel like a loophole—a way to enjoy the fizz and flavour without the glucose spike.

But are these zero-calorie sodas truly safe? Or are they just sweet illusions wrapped in clever marketing?

Let's decode what science says.

What's Really Inside a Diet Drink?

These drinks don't contain sugar, but they do contain artificial or non-nutritive sweeteners (NNS) — substances that mimic the taste of sugar without the calories. The most common ones include:

- Aspartame (found in Diet Coke, Diet Pepsi)
- Sucralose (Splenda)
- Acesulfame-K
- Saccharin
- Stevia and Monk Fruit (considered "natural" sweeteners)

They are approved by food safety bodies globally, including the FDA and FSSAI, but recent research reveals their long-term effects on blood sugar regulation, insulin sensitivity, and even gut bacteria may not be so benign.

The Metabolic Puzzle – Do Diet Drinks Really Help?

Here's where things get complicated.

1. Confuse the Brain, Confuse the Body
   Even though these sweeteners have no calories, they can still trigger a cephalic phase insulin response, where the brain, sensing sweetness, tells the pancreas to release insulin. This disconnect between taste and calories can confuse appetite regulation and fuel cravings.
2. Gut Microbiome Disruption
   Studies show artificial sweeteners like sucralose and saccharin can alter gut bacteria in ways that increase insulin resistance and glucose intolerance, even in healthy people.
3. Linked with Weight Gain – Ironically
   Multiple large-scale observational studies have found that people who regularly consume diet sodas often have higher

BMI, more belly fat, and higher diabetes risk—even though they consume fewer calories.

But Is It All Bad News?

Not necessarily. The American Diabetes Association (ADA, 2024) states that non-nutritive sweeteners can be used in moderation as a replacement for added sugars, but they are not a magic bullet. They emphasize that long-term safety data is still evolving, and these drinks shouldn't replace real lifestyle change.

The WHO (2023) went a step further—officially discouraging the use of non-sugar sweeteners for weight control or diabetes prevention, citing a lack of benefit and potential risks.

Natural vs. Artificial Sweeteners – Are They Any Better?

Stevia and Monk Fruit are often marketed as "natural" and may have fewer gut effects, but they still maintain the sweet addiction and can influence cravings.

Remember — sweet is still sweet, whether it comes from sugar or a plant.

Should Diabetics Drink Coke Zero or Diet Pepsi?

Here's the bottom line:

- Occasional use of diet drinks may be harmless—especially for people trying to wean off sugar.
- But regular, daily consumption can harm insulin sensitivity, worsen cravings, and disrupt gut health.
- Relying on them as a "safe" long-term strategy is not advisable.

What Can You Drink Instead?

Here are healthier, metabolic-friendly alternatives to quench your thirst:

- Sparkling water with a slice of lemon or cucumber
- Unsweetened herbal teas (cold or hot)
- Jeera or mint-infused water
- Buttermilk with ginger and coriander
- Homemade coconut water (in moderation)

Key Takeaway

Just because something is "zero sugar" doesn't mean it's zero risk.

As a diabetic or someone trying to improve metabolic health, it's better to reduce your sweet threshold altogether rather than substituting one addictive substance for another.

Remember: Real health doesn't come in a can.

Selected References

1. Suez J, et al. (2022). Personalized microbiome-driven effects of non-nutritive sweeteners on glucose tolerance. Cell.
2. Azad MB, et al. (2017). Nonnutritive sweeteners and cardiometabolic health: a systematic review and meta-analysis. CMAJ.
3. WHO (2023). Guideline on non-sugar sweeteners. World Health Organization.
4. Yang Q. (2010). Gain weight by "going diet?" Artificial sweeteners and the neurobiology of sugar cravings. Yale J Biol Med.

5. Pepino MY et al. (2013). Sucralose affects glycemic and hormonal responses. Diabetes Care.
6. ADA Standards of Care in Diabetes – 2024. American Diabetes Association.

CHAPTER 14

SICK-DAY RULES FOR DIABETICS – WHAT TO DO WHEN ILLNESS STRIKES

> "Fever, flu, or food poisoning—don't let them derail your sugar control."

When you have diabetes, being sick doesn't just make you feel miserable—it can push your blood sugar dangerously high or low. Whether it's a fever, infection, viral flu, or even a stomach bug, your diabetes management needs special attention during illness.

This chapter outlines the essential "sick day rules" that every person with diabetes must know to stay safe and avoid complications.

1. Why Do Blood Sugars Fluctuate When You're Sick?

- Stress hormones (like cortisol and adrenaline) are released during illness, raising blood sugar levels.

- Appetite loss and vomiting or diarrhea may lead to low blood sugar or dehydration.
- Fever, infections, or inflammation increase insulin resistance.
- Steroid medications or IV fluids can worsen hyperglycemia.

⚠ Result: Risk of diabetic ketoacidosis (DKA), especially in Type 1 diabetes, or severe hyperglycemia in Type 2.

2. Golden Sick-Day Rules

- Never stop medications without advice: Continue insulin and oral medications unless told otherwise.
- Monitor sugars frequently: Check every 4 hours or more, especially in Type 1.
- Hydration is key: Sip water, buttermilk, coconut water, or ORS every 30–60 mins.
- Watch for ketones (Type 1): Check urine or blood ketones if sugars >250 mg/dL.
- Adjust insulin as needed: May need more insulin during fever/infection (with medical advice).
- Don't skip meals completely: If not eating solids, take fluids with carbs (e.g., dal soup, rice gruel, fruit juices).
- Know when to seek help: See 'red flags' below.

3. When to Call Your Doctor Immediately 🚨

- Vomiting or diarrhea persists >6 hours.
- High fever >102°F for more than 1 day.
- Blood sugar >300 mg/dL despite insulin.
- Blood sugar <70 mg/dL and not improving with glucose.

- Positive urine or blood ketones (especially in Type 1).
- Breathing difficulty, drowsiness, or confusion.
- No urination for >8 hours (risk of dehydration and acute kidney injury).

4. **Adjusting Medications During Illness**
   - Metformin: Hold if vomiting, diarrhea, or dehydration (risk of lactic acidosis).
   - SGLT2 inhibitors (e.g., empagliflozin): Pause during fever/ infection (risk of DKA).
   - DPP-4 inhibitors (e.g., sitagliptin): Can be continued safely.
   - Sulfonylureas (e.g., glimepiride): Use cautiously if appetite is poor—risk of hypoglycemia.
   - Insulin: May need a dose increase in infection. Never skip basal insulin.

5. **Sick-Day Checklist – Keep This Handy**
   - ☑ Thermometer
   - ☑ Glucometer + test strips
   - ☑ Ketone testing strips (urine or blood)
   - ☑ Oral Rehydration Solution (ORS)
   - ☑ Ready-to-use glucose tablets or drinks
   - ☑ Contact number of your doctor or diabetes educator
   - ☑ Small frequent carb-rich fluids (e.g., soups, juices)

6. **Special Situations**
   - Diarrhea & vomiting: Use electrolyte-rich fluids like ORS. Avoid sugary sodas.

- Loss of appetite: Replace solid meals with small sips of fluids every 30–60 mins.
- Post-surgery or steroids: Monitor sugars more frequently; insulin needs may rise.
- COVID-19, dengue, or flu: Stay hydrated, avoid unmonitored over-the-counter meds.

7. **Prevent Sick Days: What You Can Do**

- Get vaccinated – annual flu, COVID boosters, pneumococcal, and hepatitis B.
- Maintain good hand hygiene and avoid close contact with infected individuals.
- Manage stress, sleep well, and ensure good nutrition for immunity.

Final Word

A single day of illness can undo months of good diabetes control—unless you're prepared. Following sick-day rules ensures that minor illnesses don't snowball into serious complications. Remember: Monitor more, hydrate often, and don't hesitate to ask for help.

References

1. American Diabetes Association. Standards of Medical Care in Diabetes – 2024.
2. IDF Clinical Practice Recommendations on the Management of Diabetes During Illness.
3. Joslin Diabetes Center. Sick-Day Guidelines for People with Diabetes.

CHAPTER 15

SHOTS THAT SHIELD – ESSENTIAL VACCINES FOR PEOPLE WITH DIABETES

Introduction

People with diabetes are more vulnerable to infections, and the outcomes are often more severe. Impaired immunity, high blood glucose, and co-existing conditions make vaccination a crucial part of diabetes care.

This chapter outlines the essential vaccines that every diabetic adult should consider, based on global and Indian guidelines.

1. Why Vaccination Is Crucial in Diabetes

- Diabetes weakens the immune response.
- Infections can worsen blood sugar control.
- Hospitalizations and complications from preventable infections are higher.

– Vaccination reduces morbidity, hospitalization, and mortality.

2. Recommended Vaccines for Adults with Diabetes (India, 2025)

- ✅ "1. Influenza (Flu) Vaccine"
  - Annual vaccine
  - Reduces flu-related hospitalizations
- ✅ "2. Pneumococcal Vaccine"
  - PCV-13 (once) + PPSV-23 (after 1 year)
  - Prevents pneumonia, bloodstream infections, meningitis
- ✅ "3. Hepatitis B Vaccine"
  - 3-dose schedule (0, 1, 6 months)
  - Risk of transmission higher in healthcare or dialysis patients
- ✅ "4. Herpes Zoster (Shingles) Vaccine"
  - Recommended above age 50
  - Prevents painful shingles outbreaks and post-herpetic neuralgia
- ✅ "5. Tdap (Tetanus, Diphtheria, Pertussis)"
  - One-time booster if not received as an adult
  - Tetanus booster every 10 years
- ✅ "6. COVID-19 Booster (as per latest variant update)"
  - Important due to increased risk of severe COVID in diabetics

3. Additional Vaccines Based on Risk

– "Hepatitis A" (if chronic liver disease or travel risk)

- "HPV" (up to age 45, especially in women)
- "Typhoid" (if traveling to endemic areas)
- "Rabies" (for occupational or pet exposure)
- "Travel vaccines" (e.g., yellow fever, cholera as per destination)

4. Vaccination Myths in Diabetics

- "Vaccines will worsen sugar levels" → No, mild fever may occur, but benefits outweigh risks.
- "I'm too old for vaccines" → Age increases risk; vaccines are more important.
- "If I missed one, I can't take the rest" → Missed doses can be caught up safely.

5. Safety Tips for Diabetic Patients

- Take vaccines when blood sugar is reasonably controlled (not during DKA or severe illness).
- Stay hydrated after shots.
- Monitor sugars more frequently for 2–3 days post-vaccination.
- Use paracetamol if mild fever or body aches occur.

Mr. Ibrahim, a retired banker with Type 2 diabetes, used to fall sick every winter. After getting his flu and pneumococcal vaccines at Satva Clinic:

- **No hospitalizations in 3 years**
- **Faster recovery from minor infections**
- **Peace of mind during COVID waves**

Mr. Ibrahim, a retired banker with Type 2 diabetes, used to fall sick every winter. After getting his flu, pneumococcal, and zoster vaccines at Satva Clinic:

- No hospitalizations in 3 years
- Faster recovery from minor infections
- Peace of mind during COVID waves

Conclusion

Vaccines are not just for children—they are shields for adults with diabetes.

By protecting yourself against preventable infections, you reduce the risk of complications, hospital stays, and even death.

"A few shots in the arm can save you a lifetime of damage."

CHAPTER 16

PERSONALIZED DIABETES – FUTURE OF GENOMICS & BIOMARKERS

> "Your DNA, your data, your diabetes plan."

We are entering an era where diabetes care is no longer just reactive—it is predictive, preventive, and profoundly personal. From decoding our genes to analyzing hormones, fat patterns, and gut microbes, modern science is reshaping how we understand and manage metabolic dysfunction.

In this chapter, we explore how emerging biomarkers and genomic insights are revolutionizing diabetes care.

1. The Genomic Revolution – What Genes Can Tell Us

- Specific gene variants affect your risk of type 2 diabetes, insulin resistance, and fat metabolism.
- Commonly studied genes:

- TCF7L2 – One of the strongest risk genes for type 2 diabetes.
- FTO – Associated with obesity and insulin resistance.
- PPARG – Involved in fat cell development and insulin sensitivity.
- SLC30A8 – Affects insulin secretion from beta cells.

– While not used for daily treatment yet, these insights can guide early lifestyle changes and medication choices in the future.

2. Toward Precision Prescriptions

– Metformin response varies with ATM and SLC22A1 gene variants.

– Sulfonylureas may work better or worse depending on KCNJ11 polymorphisms.

– Thiazolidinediones (like pioglitazone) have varying effects based on PPARG genotypes.

– Statin-induced diabetes risk may be influenced by HMGCR gene variants.

– In the future, your genetic profile may guide both drug choice and dosage.

3. Beyond Sugar: Biomarkers That Predict Before Diabetes Strikes

– Fasting Insulin and HOMA-IR: Detect insulin resistance early.

– Adiponectin and Leptin: Indicators of fat-cell dysfunction.

– High-sensitivity CRP: Marker of chronic inflammation.

- ALT, GGT, and Fatty Liver Index: Reflect liver-based insulin resistance.
- TG/HDL Ratio: A simple but powerful indicator of metabolic syndrome.
- Fasting C-peptide: Shows beta-cell function and helps tailor therapy.

4. **Your Body's Hidden Clues – Fat, Muscle, and Metabolic Risk**
   - DEXA scans and InBody analyzers reveal visceral fat %, not just BMI.
   - Higher visceral fat = higher insulin resistance, even in slim individuals (TOFI phenotype).
   - Low skeletal muscle mass worsens glucose disposal.
   - These tools personalize dietary, fitness, and medication plans beyond weight alone.

5. **Gut Microbiome Testing – The Metabolic Gatekeeper**
   - Dysbiosis (microbial imbalance) is now linked to obesity, diabetes, and inflammation.
   - Tests like GI Map, DayTwo, or Genova reveal microbial ratios, inflammation, and diversity.
   - Personalized prebiotic and probiotic recommendations are the future frontier.
   - Certain strains, like Akkermansia and Bifidobacterium are associated with better sugar control.

6. Cortisol, Chronobiology, and Stress Hormones

- Cortisol levels (morning, evening, or 24h profiles) can predict glucose spikes.
- Disrupted circadian rhythm affects insulin action and hunger hormones.
- Wearables now offer sleep stages, HRV (Heart Rate Variability), and recovery metrics.
- Personalized sleep and stress management can be as powerful as medication.

7. What's Coming: AI + Genomics + Wearables

- Labs will integrate genetic data, glucose response, inflammation, and microbiome into single dashboards.
- AI will predict disease trajectory and recommend lifestyle or drug adjustments in real time.
- Indian labs like MapmyGenome, Xcode Life, and Healthians are entering this space.
- Global leaders like ZOE, InsideTracker, and Levels are defining precision metabolic care.

Final Word

We are standing at the edge of a new era. Diabetes will no longer be diagnosed only after sugars rise, but predicted and prevented through metabolic markers, genomics, and personalized feedback loops.

The future of diabetes care is not just about lowering blood sugar—it's about decoding the unique story your body tells, and writing a healthier chapter, ahead of time.

References

1. Zeevi D, et al. Personalized Nutrition by Prediction of Glycemic Responses. Cell. 2015.
2. Franks PW, McCarthy MI. Exposing the exposures responsible for type 2 diabetes and obesity. Science. 2016.
3. Barroso I, et al. The genetic basis of metabolic disease. Cell. 2021.
4. Turnbaugh PJ, et al. The human microbiome and its potential for metabolic intervention. Nature. 2009.

SECTION 6

FINAL INSIGHTS

CHAPTER 1

THE FINAL WORD – FROM KNOWLEDGE TO ACTION

Introduction

You've just read through what most people spend decades learning the hard way. This book wasn't just about decoding diabetes—it was about reshaping how we think about health, food, and life.

Now, it's time to act. Because knowledge without action is like insulin in a vial—useless until injected into your routine.

1. The New Rules of Diabetes

- It's not just about sugar. It's about insulin resistance.
- Calories matter, but "food quality" matters more.
- Fat isn't the enemy. "Ultra-processed carbs" are.
- Exercise is medicine. So is "sleep, protein, muscle, and purpose".
- You don't need to become perfect. You need to become "consistent".

2. The Metabolic Multiplier Effect

Diabetes rarely comes alone. It walks hand-in-hand with:

- "Fatty Liver": Present in over 60% of diabetics in India.
- "PCOS": A metabolic-hormonal disorder strongly linked to insulin resistance.
- "Obstructive Sleep Apnea (OSA)": Common in overweight or obese diabetics. Poor sleep worsens sugars.
- "High Triglycerides and Hypertension": Not separate issues—they are metabolic siblings.

Treating just sugar without fixing these underlying drivers is like painting over rust.

3. The 10-Day Diabetes Reset Challenge

Here's a clinically grounded plan to start shifting your metabolism and mindset:

"● Day 1: Protein-First Breakfast"

Begin every day with a protein-based breakfast (eggs, paneer, sprouts, Greek yogurt).

[→] Lowers post-meal glucose spikes and reduces cravings throughout the day.

"● Day 2: Remove the Whites"

No sugar, maida, bread, biscuits, or white rice today.

[→] Replace with millets, dal, brown/red rice, or vegetable-based meals.

"● Day 3: Move After Meals"

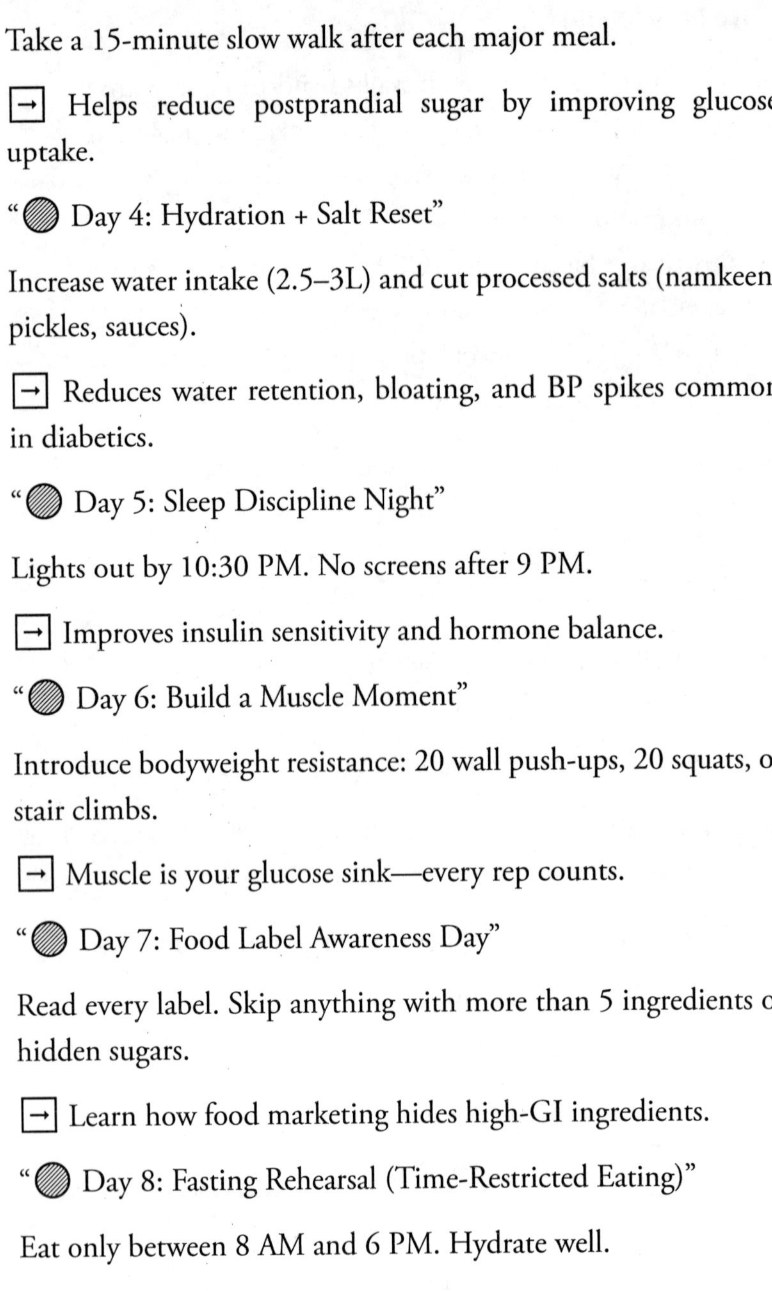

Take a 15-minute slow walk after each major meal.

→ Helps reduce postprandial sugar by improving glucose uptake.

“● Day 4: Hydration + Salt Reset”

Increase water intake (2.5–3L) and cut processed salts (namkeen, pickles, sauces).

→ Reduces water retention, bloating, and BP spikes common in diabetics.

“● Day 5: Sleep Discipline Night”

Lights out by 10:30 PM. No screens after 9 PM.

→ Improves insulin sensitivity and hormone balance.

“● Day 6: Build a Muscle Moment”

Introduce bodyweight resistance: 20 wall push-ups, 20 squats, or stair climbs.

→ Muscle is your glucose sink—every rep counts.

“● Day 7: Food Label Awareness Day”

Read every label. Skip anything with more than 5 ingredients or hidden sugars.

→ Learn how food marketing hides high-GI ingredients.

“● Day 8: Fasting Rehearsal (Time-Restricted Eating)”

Eat only between 8 AM and 6 PM. Hydrate well.

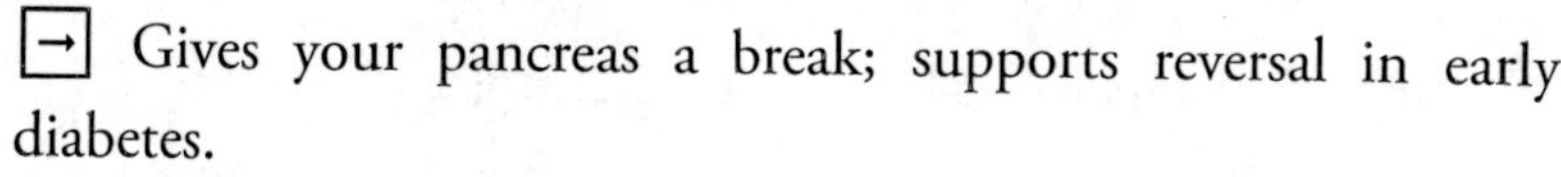

→ Gives your pancreas a break; supports reversal in early diabetes.

"◍ Day 9: Gut Health Recharge"

Include curd, fermented foods, and raw vegetable fiber today.

→ Supports microbiome diversity—linked to better glycemic control.

"◍ Day 10: Digital Detox & Reflection"

Minimal screen time. Journal 3 changes you've noticed in energy, sleep, digestion, or sugars.

→ Builds mindfulness and insight before long-term planning.

4. Purpose as the Best Medicine

Why do some patients heal faster, stick to change, and reverse diabetes—while others don't?

Because they have a "reason".
- For their children
- For their dreams
- For their faith, career, legacy

The science of "logotherapy and behavioral medicine" shows that people with a sense of purpose live longer, stick to lifestyle changes, and have lower inflammation.

5. My Closing Advice as a Physician

As someone who sees diabetes patients every day, I've learned this:
- Healing begins when people are heard, not judged.

– Your body wants to heal, but you must stop interrupting it.
– Start small. Build momentum. Let food and movement become habits, not punishments.

You're not broken. You're just misaligned. And now, you know how to realign.

Conclusion

This book may be ending, but your new chapter is just beginning.

Diabetes is not your identity. It's just your signal to wake up.

And now that you've decoded it, you can finally rewrite the script.

Let your actions become your best medicine.

CHAPTER 2

LIFESTYLE FAQS – DIABETES IN THE REAL WORLD

❓ Can Diabetics Drink Alcohol?

Yes, but with caution. Alcohol can lower blood sugar dangerously, especially when taken with insulin or sulfonylureas. Safe choices include dry wine, whiskey, or vodka in moderation—always with food and hydration.

- Never drink on an empty stomach.
- Avoid sugary cocktails and mixers.
- Monitor sugar levels before bed and the next morning.
- Avoid binge drinking or combining alcohol with SGLT2 inhibitors.

❓ Can I Eat Fruits as a Diabetic?

Fruits are naturally sweet and can spike blood sugar. Stick to:

- ✅ Avocado, Guava, Berries – safe and fiber-rich.
- ⚠ All other fruits only in very small amounts.
- ❌ Avoid mango, banana, chikoo, grapes, and fruit juices.

Best time: after meals with protein or nuts. Never on an empty stomach.

? Are Indian Spices Really Medicinal?

Yes—some spices support blood sugar and metabolic health:

- Turmeric (curcumin): anti-inflammatory and improves insulin sensitivity.
- Fenugreek (methi): reduces post-meal sugar.
- Cinnamon: may lower fasting glucose.

Use them regularly, but don't expect miracles from just one spice.

? How Safe Are Fasting Traditions?

Fasting can help reverse insulin resistance—but it must be done safely, especially during:

- Navratri, Ramadan, Jain Paryushan, or Christian Lent.

Adjust medications (especially insulin, sulfonylureas) under medical guidance. Stay hydrated. Breakfast with protein, not sweets or refined carbs.

? Which Gadgets Actually Help?

Technology can empower self-care:

- CGMs (Continuous Glucose Monitors): game-changer for sugar tracking.
- Smart watches and step counters: build accountability.
- Best Indian-friendly apps: HealthifyMe, mySugr, BeatO, Apple Health.

? Is My Gut Affecting My Diabetes?

Yes. Poor gut health (dysbiosis, low diversity) is linked to insulin resistance and inflammation.

Support gut health with:
– Curd, buttermilk, fermented foods (kanji, dosa/idli batter).
– More fiber, less sugar.
– Avoid unnecessary antibiotics.

? Can My Skin Reveal My Sugar Problem?

Absolutely. The skin gives early signs:
– Acanthosis nigricans (dark neck, armpits)
– Skin tags
– Fungal infections, dry feet, slow wound healing

If your skin speaks, listen—it often reflects internal sugar trouble.

? What Does Diabetes Reversal Really Mean?

Reversal means bringing blood sugar back to normal without the use of diabetes medications for at least 3 to 6 months.

✔ Targets:
– HbA1c < 6.5% without medication
– Fasting glucose < 100 mg/dL (ideally)
– Stable insulin and HOMA-IR levels

🔁 Don't stop medications abruptly. Work with your doctor. Reversal is real, but relapse is easy.

How Can I Protect My Feet From Diabetic Complications?

High blood sugar can damage nerves and blood vessels, causing numbness, infections, and ulcers.

Tips:
- Inspect your feet daily for cuts, color changes
- Keep feet clean, dry, and moisturized (except between toes)
- Avoid walking barefoot
- Wear soft, well-fitting footwear

Get a foot exam annually—even without symptoms.

Why Is Dental Health Important for People With Diabetes?

Gum disease (periodontitis) is more common and severe in diabetics—and it can worsen blood sugar control.

Signs to watch:
- Bleeding gums
- Bad breath
- Receding gums

Brush and floss twice a day, avoid smoking, and get dental checkups every 6 months.

What Should I Do If I Forget a Dose of My Diabetes Medication?

It depends on the medication:
- "Metformin": Take it as soon as you remember—unless it's almost time for the next dose.

- "Insulin": Check your sugar first. Missing a dose may require careful correction.
- "Sulfonylureas" (like glimepiride): Skip it if it's close to the next dose to avoid low sugar.
- "DPP-4 inhibitors" (like sitagliptin, teneligliptin): Can usually be taken later if missed.
- "SGLT2 inhibitors" (like empagliflozin): Skip the missed dose. Do not double up.

Never double your dose. Always consult your doctor if unsure.

? Is It Okay to Exercise With High Blood Sugar?

If your fasting or pre-workout sugar is "above 250 mg/dL", be cautious. Exercise may worsen hyperglycemia if insulin is deficient.

☑ If you're not feeling ill, light activity like walking may help.

✕ Avoid intense workouts until sugar stabilizes.

Always hydrate well and monitor sugar before and after workouts.

? What Should I Do in a Low Sugar Emergency (Hypoglycemia)?

Hypoglycemia means your blood sugar has dropped too low—typically below 70 mg/dL.

⚠ Symptoms include:

- Sweating
- Shakiness
- Irritability or confusion

- Rapid heartbeat
- Blurred vision or dizziness

✅ What to do immediately:

- Eat or drink "15 grams of fast-acting carbs" (e.g., 3 teaspoons sugar, 4 glucose tablets, or half a glass of fruit juice).
- Wait 15 minutes and recheck sugar.
- If still low, repeat the same.

Once sugar normalizes, follow up with a protein-rich snack (like nuts or curd).

🚑 If unconscious or unable to swallow: Do not force-feed. Seek emergency help immediately.

Always carry glucose tablets or sugar sachets if you're on insulin or sulfonylureas.